DAILY VAGUS NERVE EXERCISES

The Comprehensive Approach To Harnessing the Power of Daily Vagus Nerve Stimulation For Enhancing Mind-Body Connection, Vitality, and Inner Harmony

Julius Russel

© Copyright 2023 by Julius Russel. All rights reserved.

No portion of the 'Daily Vagus Nerve Exercises' may be replicated or disseminated in any form without the written consent of the copyright owner, Julius Russel, except for certain uses permitted under copyright law.

Table of Contents

INTRODUCTION 5

CHAPTER 1: **THE VAGUS NERVE AND ITS FUNCTIONS** 7

    THE ANATOMY AND LOCATION OF THE VAGUS NERVE 7
        Anatomy of the Vagus Nerve 7
        Branches of the Vagus Nerve 8
        Location of the Vagus Nerve 9
    ROLE OF THE VAGUS NERVE IN REGULATING THE PARASYMPATHETIC NERVOUS SYSTEM 9
    INFLUENCE OF THE VAGUS NERVE ON VARIOUS BODILY FUNCTIONS 11
    THE RELATIONSHIP BETWEEN THE VAGUS NERVE AND STRESS RESPONSE 13
        Understanding the Stress Response 13
        Role of the Vagus Nerve in the Stress Response 13

CHAPTER 2: **UNDERSTANDING THE MIND-BODY CONNECTION** 15

    THE INTRICATE CONNECTION BETWEEN THE MIND AND BODY 15
    HOW STRESS AND EMOTIONAL STATES IMPACT THE VAGUS NERVE 17
    LINK BETWEEN VAGUS NERVE HEALTH AND MENTAL WELL-BEING 18

CHAPTER 3: **BENEFITS OF DAILY VAGUS NERVE EXERCISES** 20

CHAPTER 4: **DEEP BREATHING TECHNIQUES** 23

    IMPORTANCE OF DEEP BREATHING IN ACTIVATING THE VAGUS NERVE 23
    STEP-BY-STEP INSTRUCTIONS FOR DIAPHRAGMATIC BREATHING 24
    BOX BREATHING TECHNIQUE FOR RELAXATION AND STRESS REDUCTION 25
    VARIATIONS AND MODIFICATIONS OF DEEP BREATHING EXERCISES 26

CHAPTER 5: **MEDITATION AND MINDFULNESS PRACTICES** 28

    THE IMPACT OF MEDITATION ON VAGUS NERVE STIMULATION 28
    INTRODUCTION TO DIFFERENT MEDITATION TECHNIQUES (E.G., MINDFULNESS, LOVING-KINDNESS)
   29
    TIPS FOR ESTABLISHING A REGULAR MEDITATION PRACTICE 33
    INCORPORATING MINDFULNESS INTO DAILY ACTIVITIES 35

CHAPTER 6: **THE POWER OF YOGA FOR VAGUS NERVE STIMULATION** 38

Overview Of Yoga As A Holistic Practice For Mind-Body Wellness 38

Specific Yoga Poses And Sequences That Target The Vagus Nerve 39

Incorporating Breathwork And Movement In Yoga For Vagus Nerve Activation 44

CHAPTER 7: ENGAGING THE SENSES: SOUND AND VAGUS NERVE STIMULATION 46

The Therapeutic Effects Of Sound On The Vagus Nerve 46

Using Music And Sound Therapy For Relaxation And Stress Reduction 48

Guided Auditory Exercises For Vagus Nerve Activation 49

CHAPTER 8: PHYSICAL EXERCISES AND BODYWORK 52

Understanding The Link Between Physical Activity And Vagus Nerve Function 52

Cardiovascular Exercises For Vagus Nerve Stimulation 53

Massage Techniques For Vagus Nerve Activation And Relaxation 55

CHAPTER 9: LIFESTYLE AND SELF-CARE PRACTICES FOR VAGUS NERVE HEALTH.57

Importance Of A Healthy Lifestyle In Supporting Vagus Nerve Function 57

Nutrition Tips For Optimal Vagus Nerve Health 59

Quality Sleep And Its Impact On The Vagus Nerve 61

Stress Management Techniques For Vagal Tone Enhancement 63

CHAPTER 10: BONUS: INTEGRATING VAGUS NERVE EXERCISES INTO DAILY LIFE 66

Tips For Incorporating Vagus Nerve Exercises Into A Busy Schedule 66

Strategies For Maintaining Consistency And Motivation 68

Tracking Progress And Observing The Benefits Of Regular Practice 70

CHAPTER 11: GLOSSARY OF TERMS 73

CONCLUSION 75

Introduction

Your nervous system acts as a sort of communication network, working together to bring information from the various parts of your body to the brain for processing, and then telling the body how to respond accordingly. They all have to work together, and each and every nerve serves its purpose. However, one particular nerve has made itself incredibly important. It regulates your automatic functions, keeping you alive, and ensuring that your organs are working properly. It regulates your immune system, so it is not allowed to go too far. It determines whether you are relaxed or stressed and can even be related to disorders such as depression and anxiety. This is your vagus nerve—one of the cranial nerves that travel throughout much of your body.

Your vagus nerve is believed to have three primary functions: It can allow for your body to be in connection mode, in which it is capable of facilitating a conversation with other people. It can allow for your body to be in fight or flight mode or shutdown mode in regards to how you handle stress through the use of the sympathetic and parasympathetic nervous systems. It facilitates much of your functioning that you engage in on a regular basis, and it becomes an exceedingly important factor in your life, without you ever even realizing that it is there.

Understandably, the vagus nerve has been attracting all sorts of attention lately. It is incredibly important in many different contexts of your life, and if it is not functioning properly, you can run into all sorts of problems. You can get sick more often. You can see yourself struggling with your mental health and ability to relate to other people, as well as seeing your physical health deteriorate as well. Some people have naturally low vagal tone—the measurement to determine the functionality of the vagus nerve. However, they do not have to live like this. You can tone your vagus nerve through stimulation and support that you offer to it. While doctors have been looking at methods through which you can activate and control the vagus nerve through electrical stimulation from implanted devices, you can also do so by yourself at home. You can activate your vagus nerve through activities such as moving, activating your voice, or even triggering your facial muscles.

This book is going to teach you how to do exactly that—you will learn how to stimulate and support your vagus nerve to ensure that it is functioning properly. When your vagus nerve is actively working well, you will be healthier and happier.

However, before you dive into how to stimulate the vagus nerve, you must first look at how the vagus nerve functions. You will be guided through understanding the nervous system, the vagus nerve's anatomy and interaction with the body, and how to recognize when the vagus nerve needs help. When you've finished reading this book, you'll have an excellent grasp of the significance of your vagus nerve and how to activate it in a manner that's appropriate for your needs.

It is important to keep in mind that the data contained in this book is intended solely for the intent of providing basic knowledge and isn't intended to serve as professional or medical advice. While efforts have been made to ensure the accuracy and reliability of the information,

I strongly recommend consulting with a qualified healthcare professional or specialist before implementing any of the suggestions, exercises, or practices discussed. They will be able to provide personalized advice based on your individual circumstances and medical history.

Keep in mind that each person is different and that the things which work well for some people might not work as well for others. It is essential to listen to your body, respect your limits, and seek professional guidance when necessary.

Chapter 1:

The Vagus Nerve and Its Functions

The vagus nerve, also known as the tenth cranial nerve or simply the CN X, is one of the longest and most complex nerves in the human body. It plays a vital role in the functioning of numerous organs and systems, including the parasympathetic nervous system, which controls many of the body's automatic functions.

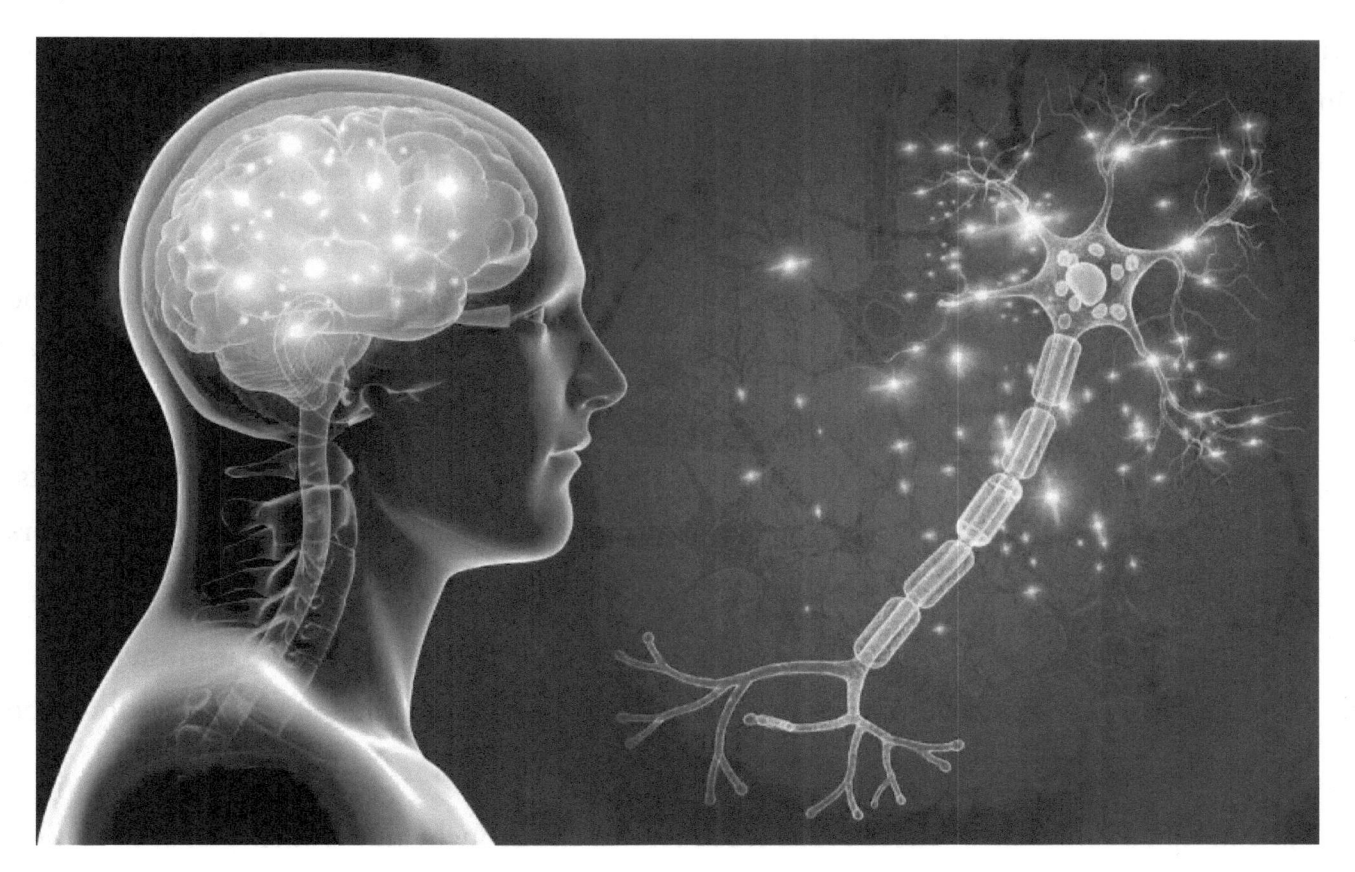

The Anatomy And Location Of The Vagus Nerve

Anatomy of the Vagus Nerve

The medulla oblongata, located at the base of the brainstem, serves as the origin of the vagus nerve. It comprises a collection of nerve fibers that emerge from the medulla and extend throughout the body. The vagus nerve is composed of a combination of motor, sensory, and autonomic fibers, granting it versatility and multiple functions.

As a component of the parasympathetic nervous system, the vagus nerve helps in regulating activities associated with rest and digestion, as well as maintaining overall balance within the body. It provides innervation to various organs and structures, including the heart, lungs, digestive system, and numerous others.

The vagus nerve exits the skull through an opening called the jugular foramen, located at the base of the skull. It then descends into the neck, where it gives off several branches and continues its course into the chest and abdomen.

Branches of the Vagus Nerve

Once the vagus nerve exits the skull, it gives rise to several important branches that innervate different structures and organs. The major branches of the vagus nerve include:

1. Pharyngeal Branches: These branches supply motor fibers to the muscles of the pharynx (throat) involved in swallowing and speaking.

2. Superior Laryngeal Nerve: This branch has both sensory and motor components. The sensory fibers provide sensory information from the larynx (voice box), while the motor fibers innervate the muscles responsible for controlling vocal cord tension.

3. Recurrent Laryngeal Nerve: This branch also has both sensory and motor components. The sensory fibers carry sensory information from the larynx, while the motor fibers innervate the muscles responsible for vocal cord movement.

4. Cardiac Branches: The vagus nerve sends branches to the heart, where it influences the heart rate and cardiac function. It provides parasympathetic innervation to slow down the heart rate and decrease cardiac contractility.

5. Pulmonary Branches: These branches innervate the bronchi and bronchioles of the lungs, playing a role in controlling the airway diameter and secretion production.

6. Esophageal Branches: The vagus nerve sends branches to the esophagus, providing motor fibers for peristalsis (muscular contractions) and sensory fibers for the perception of esophageal sensations.

7. Gastric Branches: The vagus nerve supplies motor fibers to the stomach, controlling gastric motility and acid secretion. It also carries sensory fibers, allowing us to perceive sensations like fullness or hunger.

8. Hepatic Branches: These branches innervate the liver, gallbladder, and biliary tree, contributing to the regulation of bile secretion and gallbladder contraction.

9. Intestinal Branches: The vagus nerve sends fibers to the small intestine and colon, influencing intestinal motility, blood flow, and nutrient absorption.

10. Splenic Branches: These branches innervate the spleen, playing a role in immune modulation and inflammation control.

Location of the Vagus Nerve

The vagus nerve follows a complex and extensive pathway throughout the body. After exiting the skull through the jugular foramen, it descends into the neck alongside other important structures, such as the carotid artery and internal jugular vein.

In the neck, the vagus nerve gives off its various branches, including the superior and recurrent laryngeal nerves. It continues its descent through the thorax, passing behind the root of the lung and branching into cardiac, pulmonary, and esophageal branches along the way.

As it reaches the abdomen, the vagus nerve contributes to the innervation of multiple organs, such as the stomach, liver, and intestines. It forms intricate networks and plexuses within these organs, allowing for precise control and regulation of their functions.

Notably, the vagus nerve also forms connections with other nerves and systems in the body. It communicates with the sympathetic nervous system, which is accountable for the fight-or-flight response, to maintain a balance between sympathetic and parasympathetic activity.

Overall, the vagus nerve is widely distributed and has extensive connections throughout the body. Its intricate anatomy and far-reaching innervation make it a key player in regulating numerous bodily functions and maintaining overall homeostasis.

Role Of The Vagus Nerve In Regulating The Parasympathetic Nervous System

The regulation of the parasympathetic nervous system is significantly influenced by the vagus nerve, which holds a fundamental role in this process. The parasympathetic nervous system oversees the control of various automatic functions within the body and actively facilitates a state of rest, relaxation, and restoration. To be able to gain a deeper comprehension of the complex connection that exists among the vagus nerve and the control of the parasympathetic nervous system, let's delve into the specific role that the vagus nerve plays in this intricate process.

In contrast to the sympathetic nervous system, which activates the fight-or-flight response, the parasympathetic nervous system operates in opposition to promote a state of calmness and energy conservation in the body. The vagus nerve plays a central role as the primary cranial nerve involved in carrying out parasympathetic functions throughout the body.

The vagus nerve consists of both sensory and motor fibers. The sensory fibers of the vagus nerve receive information from various organs and tissues and transmit it back to the brain for processing. On the other hand, the motor fibers of the vagus nerve transmit signals from the brain to target organs, orchestrating their activities. These motor fibers release acetylcholine, a neurotransmitter that promotes relaxation and inhibits sympathetic activity.

Here are some functions of the vagus nerve in regulating the parasympathetic nervous system:

1. **Heart Rate Regulation**

The vagus nerve assumes a critical role in regulating heart rate. It transmits parasympathetic signals to the sinoatrial (SA) node, which serves as the heart's natural pacemaker, prompting a deceleration of the heart rate. Through the release of acetylcholine, the vagus nerve diminishes the frequency and intensity of heart contractions, fostering a state of relaxation.

2. **Gastrointestinal Function**

The vagus nerve extensively innervates the gastrointestinal tract, including the esophagus, stomach, liver, pancreas, and intestines. It promotes digestion and nutrient absorption by stimulating peristalsis, which is the rhythmic contraction of the smooth muscles in the digestive system. The vagus nerve also stimulates gastric acid secretion, bile production, and pancreatic enzyme release.

3. **Respiratory Control**

The vagus nerve influences respiratory functions, particularly during rest and relaxation. It sends signals to the smooth muscles of the bronchi and bronchioles, causing them to constrict and promote airway constriction. The vagus nerve also stimulates bronchial gland secretion, which helps to keep the airways moist and protect against irritants.

4. **Regulation of Blood Pressure**

The vagus nerve contributes to maintaining blood pressure within a normal range. It achieves this by stimulating vasodilation, which is the relaxation of blood vessels, thereby reducing peripheral resistance and lowering blood pressure.

5. Control of Urinary Function

The vagus nerve influences bladder function by promoting detrusor muscle contraction (which empties the bladder) and inhibiting the internal urethral sphincter (which allows urine to flow out). This allows for proper bladder emptying and regulation of urination.

6. Control of Eye Function

The vagus nerve influences eye function through its parasympathetic control over the pupil's constriction (miosis) and the focusing ability of the lens (accommodation). These actions help to optimize visual clarity and adapt to different lighting conditions.

In addition to these functions, the vagus nerve also plays a role in modulating inflammation, immune responses, and stress responses. Its parasympathetic actions help counterbalance the sympathetic nervous system's effects, promoting a state of relaxation, rest, and restoration in the body.

Influence Of The Vagus Nerve On Various Bodily Functions

The vagus nerve, influences a wide range of bodily functions due to its extensive innervation and its role in both the parasympathetic and enteric nervous systems. Here are some of the vital bodily functions influenced by the vagus nerve:

Heart Function

The vagus nerve plays an important role in regulating heart rate and cardiac function. It provides parasympathetic innervation to the heart, which slows down the heart rate and decreases the force of cardiac contractions. The vagus nerve helps maintain a balanced and steady heart rate, promoting cardiovascular health.

Digestive System

The vagus nerve innervates various organs of the digestive system, including the esophagus, liver, stomach, pancreas, and intestines. It plays a crucial role in regulating digestion and nutrient absorption. The vagus nerve stimulates peristalsis, the coordinated contraction of smooth muscles in the digestive tract, promoting the movement of food and facilitating digestion. It also stimulates gastric acid secretion, bile production, and pancreatic enzyme release, aiding in the breakdown and absorption of nutrients.

Respiratory Function

The vagus nerve influences respiratory functions by controlling the smooth muscles of the airways. It regulates the diameter of the bronchi and bronchioles, influencing airway constriction and dilation. The vagus nerve stimulates bronchial gland secretion, which helps to keep the airways moist and protect against irritants.

Gag Reflex and Swallowing

The vagus nerve plays a role in the gag reflex, which helps prevent choking. It provides sensory innervation to the back of the throat and the soft palate, allowing the body to respond to potential threats by triggering the gag reflex. The vagus nerve is also involved in the complex process of swallowing, coordinating the movement of the muscles involved in swallowing food and liquids.

Control of Blood Pressure

The vagus nerve contributes to the regulation of blood pressure. It influences blood vessel dilation through its parasympathetic control, reducing peripheral resistance and lowering blood pressure. Additionally, the vagus nerve can sense changes in blood pressure and send feedback signals to the brain, contributing to overall blood pressure regulation.

Immune System Modulation

The vagus nerve aids in modulating the immune system's response to inflammation and infection. It releases neurotransmitters that can suppress inflammation, regulate immune cell activity, and promote immune tolerance. This interaction between the vagus nerve and the immune system is known as the "cholinergic anti-inflammatory pathway."

Stress Response and Emotional Well-being

The vagus nerve is involved in regulating the body's response to stress and promoting emotional well-being. It helps activate the relaxation response by stimulating the release of neurotransmitters, such as acetylcholine and oxytocin, which promote feelings of calmness, relaxation, and social connection.

Hormonal Regulation

The vagus nerve influences the release of various hormones in the body. It communicates with the hypothalamus, a key regulatory center in the brain, and can modulate the release of hormones involved in metabolism, appetite regulation, and stress response, such as cortisol.

Brain-Gut Axis

The vagus nerve plays a crucial role in the communication between the brain and the gut, known as the brain-gut axis. It transmits signals between the gut and the central nervous system, contributing to the regulation of gastrointestinal functions, appetite, and the perception of hunger and satiety.

Sexual Function

The vagus nerve influences sexual arousal and response. It is involved in the regulation of genital blood flow and the release of hormones and neurotransmitters associated with sexual function.

The Relationship Between The Vagus Nerve And Stress Response

The relationship between the vagus nerve and the stress response is complex and multifaceted. The vagus nerve, specifically its parasympathetic branch, plays a crucial role in modulating and regulating the body's response to stress. In this section, we will explore the connection between the vagus nerve and the stress response in detail.

Understanding the Stress Response

Stress is a physiological and psychological response to challenging or threatening situations. When the body perceives a threat, whether real or imagined, it activates the stress response to prepare for a fight-or-flight reaction. Cortisol and adrenaline are two examples of the stress hormones that are released in reaction to this stimulus, and triggers various physiological changes to increase alertness, energy, and readiness to respond.

The stress response is primarily mediated by the sympathetic nervous system, which prepares the body for immediate action. It leads to improved heart rate, elevated blood pressure, enhanced muscle tension, and heightened mental alertness. However, a balanced stress response also requires the involvement of the parasympathetic nervous system, in which the vagus nerve plays a crucial role.

Role of the Vagus Nerve in the Stress Response

The vagus nerve, an important constituent of the parasympathetic nervous system, is commonly known as the "rest-and-digest" or "calm-and-connect" system. Its role is complementary to that of the sympathetic nervous system, which triggers the stress response.

In times of stress, the vagus nerve acts as a regulatory mechanism, applying a brake to the stress response and aiding in the restoration of balance and relaxation. It counteracts the effects of the sympathetic nervous system and facilitates the body's return to a state of calm and equilibrium. The vagus nerve achieves this through several mechanisms:

- Activation of the Relaxation Response: The vagus nerve stimulates the release of acetylcholine, a neurotransmitter that promotes relaxation and inhibits sympathetic activity. Acetylcholine acts as a calming agent, counterbalancing the effects of stress hormones. Activation of the vagus nerve triggers a cascade of relaxation responses, including reduced heart rate, lowered blood pressure, and relaxed muscles.
- Inhibition of the HPA Axis: The HPA axis is a key hormonal system involved in the stress response. The vagus nerve helps regulate the HPA axis by inhibiting the release of stress hormones, like cortisol, from the adrenal glands. By dampening the HPA axis activity, the vagus nerve helps prevent the excessive and prolonged release of stress hormones, which can have detrimental effects on health.
- Modulation of Inflammation: Chronic stress can lead to systemic inflammation, which is associated with various health conditions. The vagus nerve plays a role in modulating inflammation through its interaction with the immune system. It releases neurotransmitters that can suppress inflammation, reduce the production of pro-inflammatory cytokines, and promote anti-inflammatory processes. This anti-inflammatory effect of the vagus nerve contributes to the overall regulation of the stress response.
- Regulation of Heart Rate Variability (HRV): Heart rate variability refers to the variation in time intervals amongst consecutive heartbeats. Higher HRV is associated with better stress resilience and adaptability. The vagus nerve influences HRV by exerting parasympathetic control over the heart. It helps maintain a balanced autonomic nervous system by increasing parasympathetic tone, resulting in increased HRV. Higher HRV indicates a flexible and adaptable stress response.
- Emotional Regulation: The vagus nerve is involved in regulating emotions and promoting emotional well-being. It influences the release of neurotransmitters, like serotonin and oxytocin, which are involved in mood regulation and social bonding. Activation of the vagus nerve can promote positive emotions, reduce anxiety and depression, and enhance social connection.

Chapter 2:

Understanding the Mind-Body Connection

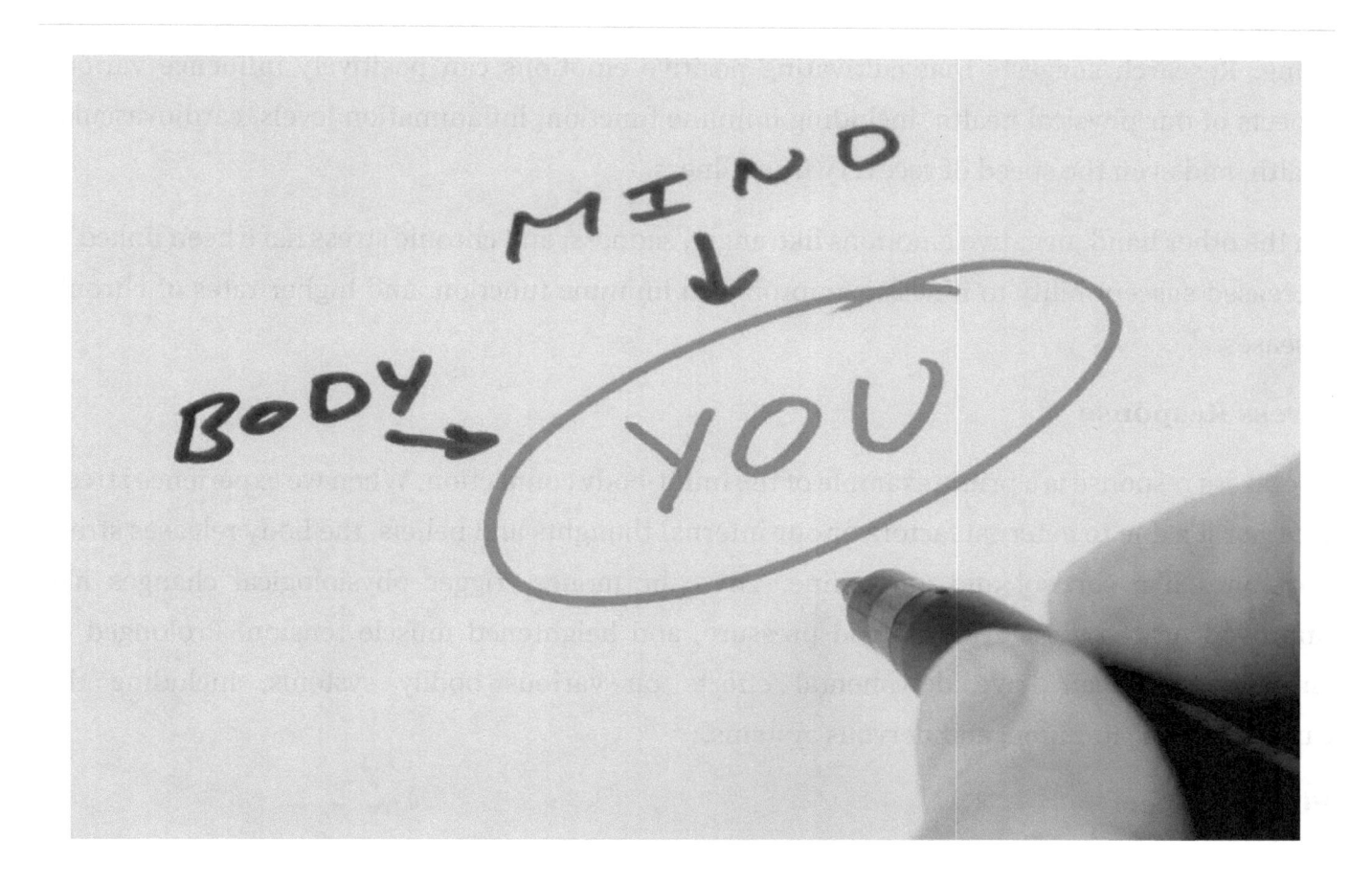

The Intricate Connection Between The Mind And Body

The interaction that exists among our thoughts, feelings, and beliefs, as well as our physical health, is referred to as the mind-body connection. Research has shown that the mind and body are not distinct things but rather intertwined aspects that significantly impact each other. Here, we will explore the intricate connection between the mind and body and how they influence one another.

Psychosomatic Influence

The mind has a profound influence on the body, and psychological factors can manifest as physical symptoms. Stress, anxiety, and emotional distress can manifest as physical ailments such as headaches, muscle tension, digestive issues, and cardiovascular problems. This phenomenon is known as psychosomatic symptoms, where emotional or psychological factors contribute to physical symptoms. It highlights how our mental state can directly impact our physical well-being.

Emotional Impact on Health

Our emotional well-being has a profound impact on our physical health. Positive emotions, such as happiness, joy, and love, have been shown to have significant benefits for our overall well-being. Research suggests that cultivating positive emotions can positively influence various aspects of our physical health, including immune function, inflammation levels, cardiovascular health, and even the speed of recovery from illness.

On the other hand, negative emotions like anger, sadness, and chronic stress have been linked to increased susceptibility to illness, compromised immune function, and higher rates of chronic diseases.

Stress Response

The stress response is a prime example of the mind-body connection. When we experience stress, whether it's due to external factors or our internal thoughts and beliefs, the body releases stress hormones like cortisol and adrenaline. These hormones trigger physiological changes like improved heart rate, elevated blood pressure, and heightened muscle tension. Prolonged or chronic stress can have detrimental effects on various bodily systems, including the cardiovascular, immune, and nervous systems.

Placebo Effect

The placebo effect demonstrates the power of the mind in influencing the body. Placebos are inactive substances or treatments that have no physiological effect, yet they can produce significant improvements in symptoms or even lead to actual physiological changes. The placebo effect highlights how our beliefs, expectations, and perceptions can influence our physical health and well-being.

Mind-Body Interventions

Various mind-body interventions, such as meditation, yoga, mindfulness, and relaxation techniques, have been shown to positively impact physical health. These practices help reduce stress, enhance emotional well-being, and promote relaxation, leading to improvements in cardiovascular health, immune function, pain management, and overall quality of life. These interventions work by harnessing the mind's power to influence the body's physiological processes.

Neuroplasticity

The capability of the brain to adapt and reorganize its structure as a result of new encounters and new ways of thinking is referred to as neuroplasticity. Our thoughts, beliefs, and behaviors can shape the structure and functioning of our brains. Positive thoughts and practices that promote well-being can strengthen neural pathways associated with resilience, emotional regulation, and cognitive flexibility. On the other hand, negative thoughts and patterns can reinforce neural pathways associated with stress, anxiety, and depression.

Gut-Brain Axis

The gut-brain axis highlights the bidirectional communication between the gut and the brain. The gut, frequently discussed as the "second brain," comprises a complex network of neurons that communicate with the central nervous system. The gut microbiota, the trillions of microorganisms residing in the gut, also play a crucial role in this communication. Research suggests that disruptions in the gut-brain axis can contribute to numerous mental health conditions, like anxiety, depression, and even neurodegenerative disorders.

Mind-Body Techniques in Healthcare

Mind-body techniques are increasingly being integrated into healthcare settings to complement traditional medical approaches. Practices like CBT, MBSR, and integrative medicine combine psychological and physical approaches to promote holistic health and well-being. These approaches recognize the interconnectedness of the mind and body and the importance of addressing both aspects for optimal health outcomes.

How Stress And Emotional States Impact The Vagus Nerve

The vagus nerve has another important role: The management of emotions and stress. Emotions are difficult to navigate because they are primarily entirely irrational. There is nothing rational about your feelings of happiness—they are simply gut responses, so to speak. You have emotions to help you navigate through your world. They are primarily meant to be motivating for you in hopes of having you instinctively do the right thing. For example, when you feel afraid, you respond by running away or avoiding the threat because you know that it is a threat, and you need to avoid it. This is meant to keep you alive. However, if you feel disgusted by something, you know that you cannot eat it for some reason—usually, because something about it is repulsive enough for you to avoid it entirely.

This is normal and makes perfect sense—you are still inherently an animal, and animals are inherently reactionary. This is not a fault with you, but rather something that you must be willing and able to consider and recognize. Your emotions are going to arise, whether you want them or not. However, you can learn how to regulate them.

Your vagus nerve plays a role in the social nervous system—that feeling of calmness when you are in that rest and digest activation of the parasympathetic nervous system. This is when you are able to connect with people and really relate to them. This is the state that you want to be in if you are going to be considering emotional regulation. This is associated with a good balance between your systems.

Sometimes, of course, you see activation from other areas of the vagus nerve instead. When the sympathetic nervous system is active, you are going to see activity within the individual in general. It can be seen as anxiety and anger, and will oftentimes be related to all of this. Your sympathetic nervous system, when in control, is likely to lead to all sorts of negativity. Especially when the sympathetic nervous system picks up on the potential threat or danger, it can quickly turn into a fight or flight response. You must remember, however, that the sympathetic activation when in a social mood can actually lead toward playing and constructive interactions as well.

Finally, the parasympathetic activation will lead to relaxation. It will usually lead to relaxation and other good feelings and desires, such as bonding with people and relaxing. However, if in the parasympathetic activation, you are threatened, or your body turns into the tendency to withdraw. It can even lead to depression if not managed at all, and that is a problem for most people.

Link Between Vagus Nerve Health And Mental Well-Being

One of the primary ways in which the vagus nerve influences mental well-being is through its role in regulating emotions and stress. It is involved in the modulation of the stress response by inhibiting the release of stress hormones, like cortisol, from the adrenal glands. By dampening the stress response, the vagus nerve helps prevent the excessive and prolonged activation of the sympathetic nervous system, which can contribute to anxiety, depression, and other mental health conditions.

Moreover, the vagus nerve is connected to various brain regions involved in emotional regulation, including the amygdala and prefrontal cortex. Through these connections, the vagus nerve influences emotional responses, helping to regulate and modulate the intensity of emotions. Individuals with higher vagal tone, which refers to the strength and efficiency of the vagus nerve, tend to have better emotional regulation and are more resilient to stress.

The vagus nerve assumes a crucial function in the body's regulation of inflammation. Chronic inflammation is linked to an elevated susceptibility to mental health disorders like depression and anxiety. Through its ability to suppress the production of pro-inflammatory cytokines and facilitate anti-inflammatory processes, the vagus nerve contributes to a more balanced and healthier inflammatory response. By modulating inflammation, the vagus nerve may indirectly impact mental well-being.

Furthermore, the vagus nerve is involved in the regulation of the autonomic nervous system, which controls various involuntary bodily functions. This includes heart rate variability (HRV), which states to the variation in time intervals amongst successive heartbeats. Higher HRV is associated with better stress resilience and adaptability. The vagus nerve influences HRV by increasing parasympathetic tone, leading to increased variability in heart rate. Higher HRV is linked to improved mental well-being, cognitive function, and emotional regulation.

Research has also suggested a potential link between vagus nerve stimulation and improvements in mental health conditions. Vagus nerve stimulation (VNS) is a therapeutic technique that comprises delivering electrical impulses to the vagus nerve, typically through an implantable device. VNS has been used as a treatment option for certain mental health disorders, including treatment-resistant depression and epilepsy. While the precise mechanisms underlying the therapeutic effects of VNS are not fully understood, it is thought to modulate neural circuits involved in mood regulation and improve overall brain function.

Chapter 3:

Benefits of Daily Vagus Nerve Exercises

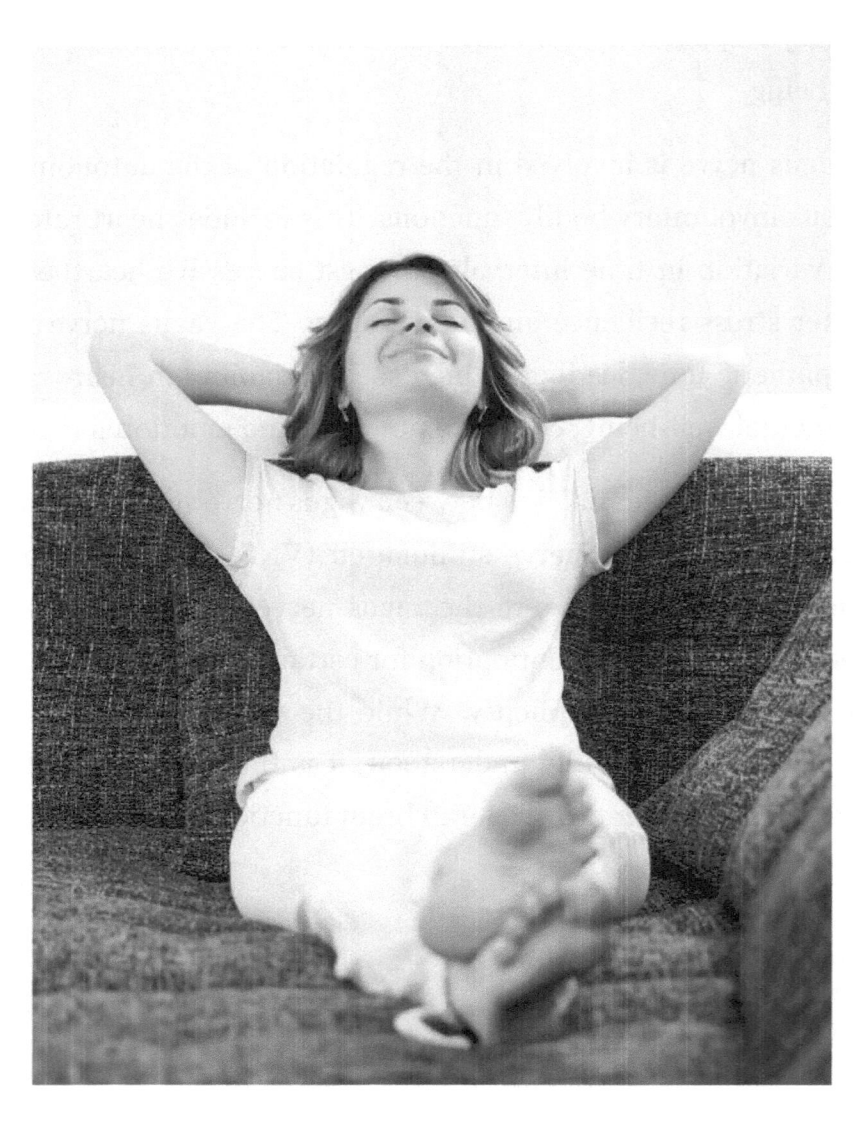

Incorporating daily vagus nerve exercises into your routine can provide a multitude of benefits for your overall health and well-being. By engaging in these exercises regularly, you can experience the following advantages:

Stress Reduction and Relaxation

Daily vagus nerve exercises activate the parasympathetic nervous system, which promotes relaxation and counters the body's stress response. By engaging in techniques such as deep breathing, meditation, or yoga, you can stimulate the vagus nerve and trigger the release of neurotransmitters that induce a state of calmness, reducing stress levels and promoting overall relaxation.

Improved Digestion and Gut Health

The vagus nerve helps in regulating digestive functions, including the production of stomach acid, enzyme secretion, and intestinal motility. Regular vagus nerve exercises can enhance these processes, leading to improved digestion and nutrient absorption. Additionally, a healthy vagus nerve supports a balanced gut microbiota, contributing to better gut health and reducing the risk of gastrointestinal disorders.

Enhanced Immune System Function

Activation of the vagus nerve has been shown to modulate the immune response, influencing the release of anti-inflammatory substances and promoting immune system balance. Daily vagus nerve exercises help regulate immune system function, leading to improved defense against infections, reduced inflammation, and better overall immune health.

Emotional Regulation and Increased Resilience

The vagus nerve is involved in regulating emotions and is connected to various brain regions associated with emotional processing. Regular stimulation of the vagus nerve through exercises can enhance emotional regulation, helping individuals better cope with stress, manage anxiety and depression, and increase resilience in the face of challenges. This benefit is attributed to the vagus nerve's influence on neurotransmitters, such as serotonin and dopamine, which are crucial for mood regulation.

Improved Heart Health

Daily vagus nerve exercises, such as deep breathing, can enhance heart rate variability (HRV), which refers to the variation in time intervals amongst heartbeats. Increased HRV is associated with better cardiovascular health, reduced risk of heart disease, and improved overall heart function.

Enhanced Cognitive Function

Activation of the vagus nerve has been linked to enhanced cognitive performance, including attention, memory, and information processing. Regular vagus nerve exercises, such as meditation and deep breathing, can increase blood flow and oxygenation to the brain, supporting cognitive function and mental clarity. These exercises also promote neuroplasticity, the brain's ability to adapt and form new connections, which is crucial for learning and memory.

Alleviation of Anxiety and Depression

Daily vagus nerve exercises can have a positive impact on mental health. By stimulating the vagus nerve, these exercises promote the release of neurotransmitters, like serotonin and gamma-aminobutyric acid (GABA), which are involved in mood regulation. This can lead to reduced anxiety and depressive symptoms, promoting a greater sense of well-being.

Better Sleep Quality

The relaxation and stress reduction effects of vagus nerve exercises can positively impact sleep quality. By promoting a calm state of mind and reducing stress levels, these exercises can help individuals fall asleep faster, experience fewer sleep disturbances, and enjoy more restful and rejuvenating sleep.

Pain Management

Vagus nerve stimulation through exercises has shown potential in managing chronic pain conditions. By triggering the body's natural pain-modulating mechanisms, such as the release of endorphins and the reduction of inflammatory markers, daily vagus nerve exercises can help alleviate pain symptoms and improve pain management.

Enhanced Respiratory Function

The vagus nerve has a direct influence on respiratory muscles and lung function. Daily exercises that involve deep breathing can help strengthen respiratory muscles, improve lung capacity, and promote efficient oxygen exchange. This can enhance overall respiratory health and contribute to a sense of vitality and well-being.

Positive Mood and Emotional Well-being

Regular vagus nerve exercises can positively impact mood and emotional well-being. The stimulation of the vagus nerve promotes the release of neurotransmitters and hormones associated with positive emotions, such as dopamine and oxytocin. This can lead to an uplifted mood, increased feelings of happiness, and overall emotional well-being.

Improved Social Connections

The vagus nerve is involved in social engagement and the formation of social bonds. By promoting emotional regulation and reducing stress, daily vagus nerve exercises can enhance social interactions, communication, and the ability to connect with others on a deeper level.

Chapter 4:

Deep Breathing Techniques

Importance Of Deep Breathing In Activating The Vagus Nerve

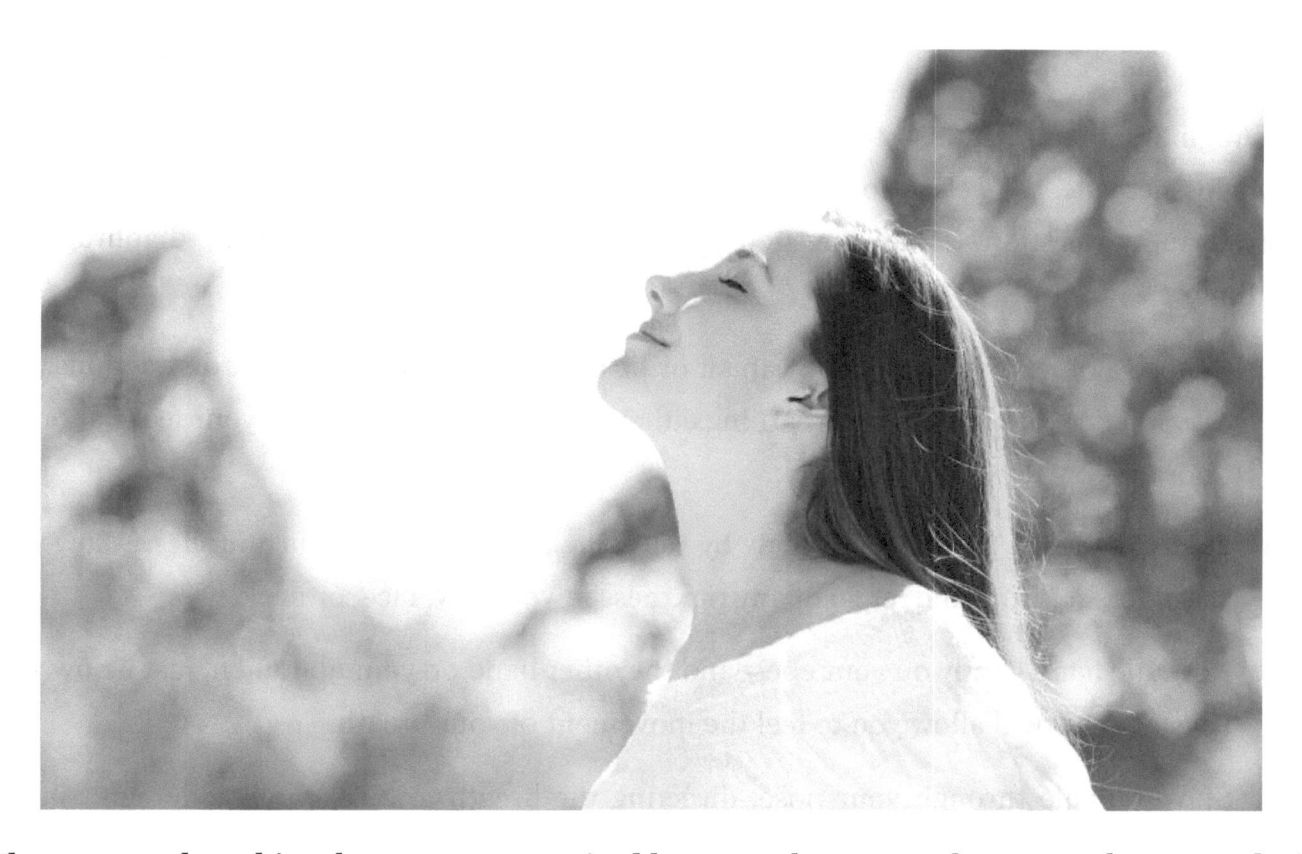

When you are breathing, have you ever noticed how your heart rate changes? When you take in a deep breath, you may feel your pulse quicken, and as you exhale, you notice it drop again. This is for a very specific reason—your vagus nerve is regulating your heart rate. When you breathe in, you trigger your pulse to quicken, and as your pulse quickens, it raises blood pressure.

That raise in blood pressure and pulse triggers your parasympathetic nervous system to kick in—it wants to regulate your heart rate, so it dumps some acetylcholine into your blood stream, slowing the heart rate. This is important to keep in mind—it means that you can effectively kick your vagus nerve into action simply by taking a deep breath in and cuing to the nerve that you are in need of some regulation to keep your heart rate steady. Your vagus nerve, as you exhale, is at its most active, slowing your heart rate the most. This means, then, that you are able to effectively regulate yourself and your parasympathetic nervous system all through breathing.

This is nothing new—in fact, the breathing pattern that triggers this state of calmness thanks to the parasympathetic nervous system actually arises in several different calming, spiritual activities. Mantras used during any sort of meditation can trigger this sort of activation, creating the proper timing between breaths and holding them, as do saying the Ave Maria prayer. The breathing rate during these techniques is dropped down to about six breaths every minute, which is what these breathing techniques will aim for.

Step-By-Step Instructions For Diaphragmatic Breathing

Diaphragmatic breathing, also referred to as belly breathing or deep breathing, is a technique that helps activate the relaxation response and engage the diaphragm, the primary muscle involved in respiration. Here are step-by-step instructions for practicing diaphragmatic breathing:

1. Choose a quiet area where you can sit or lie down comfortably without distractions. You can practice diaphragmatic breathing either in a seated position with your feet flat on the floor or lying down on your back.

2. Take a moment to relax your body by releasing any tension in your muscles. Allow your shoulders to drop, and let go of any tightness in your jaw, face, or neck.

3. Rest one hand gently on your chest and the other hand on your abdomen, just below your ribcage. This will allow you to feel the movement of your breath.

4. Slowly inhale through your nose, directing the breath towards your abdomen. As you breathe in, feel your abdomen rise, allowing it to expand fully as you fill your lungs with air. Your chest should rise only slightly, while the primary movement should be in your abdomen.

5. Slowly exhale through your mouth, focusing on fully emptying your lungs. As you exhale, feel your abdomen gently contract and sink back towards your spine.

6. Inhale deeply through your nose, feeling your abdomen expand, and exhale slowly through your mouth, feeling your abdomen contract. Take your time with each breath, allowing the inhalation and exhalation to be slow, smooth, and controlled.

7. Practice diaphragmatic breathing at a pace that feels comfortable for you. There is no need to rush or force the breath. Aim for a smooth and relaxed rhythm.

8. While maintaining a steady and deep breathing pattern, shift your focus towards the physical experience of your breath. Observe the gentle expansion and contraction of your abdomen as you inhale and exhale. You can also count the duration of your inhalation and exhalation to help maintain a steady rhythm.

9. You should begin by using diaphragmatic breathing for a couple of mins, and then progressively extend the amount of time you do it as you feel more relaxed. You can practice this technique for 5 to 10 minutes or longer, depending on your preference.

10. Make diaphragmatic breathing a regular part of your daily routine. You can practice it in the morning to start your day with a sense of calm, during stressful moments to reduce anxiety, or before bed to promote relaxation and better sleep.

Box Breathing Technique For Relaxation And Stress Reduction

Box breathing, additionally referred to as square breathing or four-square breathing, is a simple yet powerful approach for relaxation and stress reduction. Other names for box breathing are four-square breathing and square breathing. It comprises consciously controlling your breath in a specific pattern to promote a sense of calm and balance in your body and mind. This technique is widely used in various practices such as yoga, meditation, and mindfulness.

Steps:

1. To begin, locate a position that feels comfortable for you, whether it's sitting or lying down. Ensure that your spine is straight and your body is relaxed. You may choose to close your eyes to enhance your focus and minimize distractions.

2. Take a moment to bring your attention to your breath. Notice the natural rhythm of your breath without attempting to change it. Observe the sensation of the breath as it enters and leaves your body.

3. Begin the box breathing technique by inhaling slowly and deeply through your nose. Imagine filling your abdomen, then your lower chest, and finally your upper chest with the breath. Allow your breath to be smooth and effortless. As you inhale, count to four in your mind.

4. Once you have completed the inhalation, hold your breath for a count of four. During this phase, maintain a sense of stillness and relaxation in your body. If holding your breath for

four counts feels uncomfortable, you can start with a shorter duration and gradually increase it as you become more comfortable.

5. Release the breath slowly and completely through your mouth. Again, count to four in your mind as you exhale. Allow any tension or stress to leave your body with each breath. Feel the relaxation and release as you empty your lungs.

6. After exhaling, hold your breath for a count of four. Maintain a sense of calm and stillness during this pause. Use this time to settle into the present moment and embrace the sensation of being fully present.

7. Repeat the cycle of box breathing by taking another inhalation for the count of four, keeping the breath for the same number of counts, releasing for the same number of counts, and then taking another inhalation for the same number of counts. Keep up this rhythm for many mins or till you experience a sensation of peace and tranquility coming over you, whichever comes first.

Variations And Modifications Of Deep Breathing Exercises

While there are various techniques for deep breathing, it's important to note that individual preferences and needs may vary. Fortunately, there are several variations and modifications of deep breathing exercises that can be tailored to suit different situations and personal preferences. Aside from diaphragmatic and box breathing, we will discuss some other common variations and modifications of deep breathing exercises.

1. **4-7-8 Breathing Technique**

The 4-7-8 breathing technique, developed by Dr. Andrew Weil, is a simple and effective variation of deep breathing that involves a specific breath-holding pattern. This technique can be helpful for relaxation, stress reduction, and aiding with sleep. Here's how to practice the 4-7-8 breathing technique:

- Discover a comfortable position and relax your body.
- While keeping a low profile, inhale calmly via your nose for a count of four in your head.
- Stop breathing until the count of seven has passed.
- Allow all of your breath escape via your mouth as you count to eight, generating a "whooshing" sound as you do so.
- You will take an overall of four breaths if you repeat the procedure a further three times. The 4-7-8 breathing technique helps to regulate the breath, slow down the heart rate, and induce a sense of relaxation and calm.

2. **Alternate Nostril Breathing**

Alternate nostril breathing is a yogic breathing technique that balances the flow of breath and energy in the body. This technique can help to harmonize the nervous system, improve focus, and bring about a sense of balance. Here's how to practice alternate nostril breathing:

- Use your ring finger to gently close your left nostril, blocking the airflow.
- Exhale fully and completely through your right nostril, allowing the breath to flow out smoothly.
- Next, inhale deeply and slowly through your right nostril, feeling the air entering your body.
- Once you've completed the inhalation, use your thumb to close your right nostril, temporarily blocking the airflow.
- Release your ring finger from your left nostril then exhale gradually and completely through your left nostril.
- After the exhalation, inhale deeply and slowly through your left nostril.
- Once you've finished the inhalation, close your left nostril again with your ring finger.
- Release your thumb from your right nostril, allowing you to exhale through your right nostril.
- Repeat these steps, alternating between closing the left and right nostrils for inhalation and exhalation.

3. **Visualization and Affirmation**

Another modification of deep breathing exercises involves incorporating visualization and affirmation techniques. This involves combining deep breathing with positive imagery and affirmations to enhance the relaxation response and promote a positive mindset. Here's how to incorporate visualization and affirmation into your deep breathing practice:

- Choose a posture that is suitable for you, and then rest your entire body.
- Start by taking a few slow, deep breaths while focusing on the feeling of air entering and exiting your body with each inhalation.
- As you continue to breathe deeply, visualize a peaceful scene or a place that brings you joy and relaxation. Imagine yourself being present in that scene, taking in the sights, sounds, and sensations.
- While maintaining the deep breathing rhythm, repeat positive affirmations or mantras in your mind. These affirmations can be personalized statements that promote relaxation, self-confidence, or well-being.
- Continue this practice for several minutes, allowing the combination of deep breathing, visualization, and affirmations to bring about a sense of calm and positivity. Visualization and affirmation techniques add a cognitive component to deep breathing exercises, amplifying their effects on the mind and promoting a positive mental state.

Chapter 5:
Meditation and Mindfulness Practices

The Impact Of Meditation On Vagus Nerve Stimulation

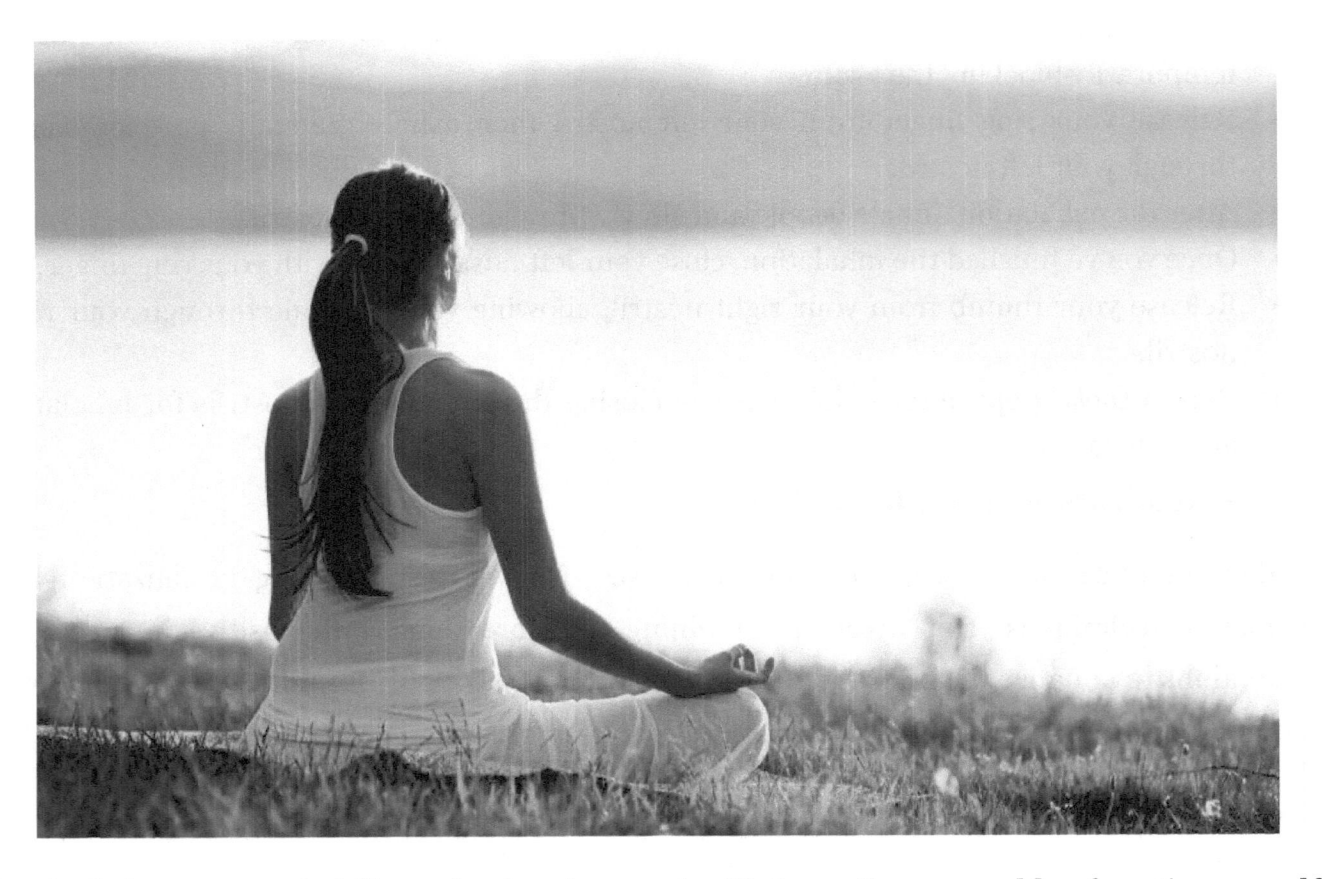

Our body has a natural ability to heal and renew itself. Our cells are capable of continuous self-repair and regeneration. Imagine if all the zits, wounds, and scrapes you have had since infancy had not healed and you were covered in bruises and dents; not a very good picture is it? It is important to understand that our internal organs are susceptible to wear and tear, as well. This means that the body's self-healing mechanism is necessary in keeping cells renewed and in a functional state at all times.

The body's self-healing mechanism is driven by the autonomic nervous system, which facilitates the parasympathetic and sympathetic responses. Sympathetic responses are our bodies' way of responding to threats and stresses. Are you running from a burning building? Are you stressed?

Anxious? In all these situations, the sympathetic nervous system is activated and in order to facilitate the fight or flight responses that we need to resolve the threats in our environment.

Consider a situation where the sympathetic system did not kick in when you were facing an imminent threat. There you are, watching this huge dog charging you, and all you can do is stand there transfixed with mouth agape. When you visualize that kind of scenario, it becomes apparent why we need these sympathetic responses. Without them, we would be vulnerable to every danger and threat that comes our way.

The downside to this system, however, is that your nervous system cannot differentiate between when you are being chased by an actual tiger or when you are freaking out over not being able to fit into your favorite pants. As far as the nervous system is concerned, these situations are both threats, and the response elicited is the same, which is basically to switch on the fight or flight responses.

When this happens, the body directs all its energies to functions that are required for fight or fleeing, including increasing the heartbeat to supply more oxygen to the muscles. While this is going on, the body's self-healing mechanism is inhibited and cannot take place until the body reverts to a restive state.

Stress kills, and it does so by impacting on your physical health as well as your psychological state. The fact of the matter is every time you are anxious, depressed, worried, or agitated, your body's self-healing mechanisms are switched off as your body primes itself to either flee or fight the threats you are facing. So, if you want to restore the body's ability to heal itself, what should you do? Well, it's pretty simple; find a means to manage stress and anxiety and activate your vagus nerve in the process.

Living your life trying to avoid pain and stress would be an exercise in futility because while you can control your own actions, you cannot control what others do. Learning to handle stress is a sure way to a healthier body and mind. Fortunately, there are various methods that we can use in destressing and attaining inner peace irrespective of what is going on around us. One of the best techniques for achieving inner peace and mindfulness is meditation.

Introduction To Different Meditation Techniques (E.G., Mindfulness, Loving-Kindness)
Mindfulness Meditation

In mindful meditation, the goal is typically to concentrate your mind on the thoughts, sensations, and emotions that you are experiencing in the present or current moment. It normally involves regulation of breathing, muscle and body relaxation, mental visualization, and a heightened awareness of the body and mind.

Mindfulness meditation is effective in stress reduction, cognitive therapy, as well as in the treatment of depression symptoms. The basic technique involved is easy to learn and can easily be done for about 10 minutes daily to obtain the benefits in terms of increasing your vagal tone.

A simple mindful meditation technique for beginners is described below:

- Find a quiet and well-aerated room to practice your meditation in.
- Sit comfortably on a chair, or you can sit on the floor.
- Make sure that your posture is relaxed and that your shoulder and neck muscles are not tense.
- Your head, neck, and spine should be aligned but not tense or stiff.
- Bring your mind to the present by pulling all your focus to the here and now.
- Concentrate on your breathing, feel the breath enter your body as you inhale, and feel the air exit your body as you exhale.
- Take deep breaths all the time, concentrating on the sensation of the rising and falling of your diaphragm.
- To make it easier to focus on your breathing, you can place one hand on your upper chest and the other above your navel. This will aid you in engaging your diaphragm when breathing in and out.
- Breath in slowly through your nose, as you inhale, the hand on your navel area should feel your stomach rise gradually as the air enters your body.
- On the exhale, let the breath out through your mouth with your lips slight pursued. As you exhale, the hand on the navel area should feel the stomach relax and fall back into the starting position.
- As thoughts pop up in your mind, do not quash or try to suppress them; simply turn your attention back to your breathing and focus on the inhale and exhale motions of rising and falling.
- Stay in this state for at least 10 minutes, always pulling your focus back to the present and away from thoughts and emotions by simply focusing on your breathing.
- At the end of the 10 minutes, rise slowly from your position, and allow your mind to become gradually aware of your surroundings.

When you become good at this type of meditation through repeated practice, you will be able to practice mindful meditation without necessarily having to find a quiet room or sit on the floor. The main aim of mindful meditation is to increase your awareness of the present moment by focusing your attention on the now and ignoring thoughts and emotions.

The effect of mindful meditation on your vagal tone is powerful because by reducing stress and inhibiting flight and fight responses that are activated when we are anxious or worried, it allows the body to relax and rest which is the ideal condition for the parasympathetic system to function. Mindful meditation has been found to be effective in reducing inflammation and improving stress resilience.

More benefits of mindful meditation include:

- Increased self-awareness
- Improved concentration and cognitive aptitude
- Better emotional regulation and management
- The overall reduction in stress and anxiety.

Breath Awareness Meditation

Breath awareness meditation is similar to mindfulness meditation in that it encourages you to focus on your breathing as a way of soothing and calming your body. The goal in breath awareness meditation is to concentrate on the breathing motions and sensations and ignore any thought that may crop up in your mind.

A simple technique to follow for this type of meditation involves following the steps outlined below:

- This meditation can be done in an upright or sitting position or even laying down on your back
- You can do this with your eyes closed, or you can leave them open, but your gaze should be down and not looking at anything in particular.
- Feel the muscles on your shoulders the back of your head and neck area. Focus your attention on these three areas.
- Breath in slowly through your nostrils and feel the rise of your shoulders as the air is getting into your body.
- Exhale slowly, and this time, focus on the falling of your shoulders as the breath leaves your body.
- With each inhaling and exhaling action, feel your jaw, shoulders, and neck beginning to loosen up and relax.
- Upon taking some breaths inhaling and exhaling, I start to realize that I am exhaling when I am supposed to be inhaling. Again, the point of this is to ensure that your mind is entirely focused on your breathing.
- Continue to monitor your breathing for about ten minutes.

- As you come towards the end of the ten minutes, you can stop thinking I am breathing out with the inhale and I am breathing out with the exhale. Allow your mind to stray from the concentration on the breathing.
- While you are exiting this focused concentration on the breathing, ask yourself, "What do I want?" on the inhale and listen to the response from your mind on the exhale.
- Then on the next inhale, ask yourself, "What am I thankful for?' and listen for the answer in your mind as you exhale.
- Acknowledge what you are you are feeling at that moment, open your eyes or bring your gaze back up, and rise from your meditation position.

Body Scan Meditation

Body scan meditation primarily involves examining or scanning your body for areas of tension. The aim is to identify areas where your muscles are tensed or where you have tension knots and essentially relax them to release the tension. The general technique in body scan meditation involves scanning your body from one end to the other. For instance, you can start from toe to head. The following steps can help you in practicing body scan meditation:

- Sit in a comfortable position and relax your body.
- Slow your breathing drown and focus on deep breathing, which is breathing from your stomach, not your chest.
- To help you in breathing from the belly, you can create a mental image of a balloon inflating and deflating in your stomach as you breath in and out.
- Focus on each part of your body, and feel for signs of tension, start from your head and work yourself down systematically through the neck chest abdomen and limbs.
- During this systematic scanning process, keep doing your deep breathing as it will heighten your awareness and ability to detect tension in your muscles.
- Notice the general feeling and sensations in different parts of your body, for instance, if you have soreness, tightness, or tense muscles in any part of your body.
- Once you come across the areas on the body that is tense or uncomfortable, focus on this area as you breathe in and out. You can accompany this focus by gently massaging the area of tension and concentrate on feeling the tension leave your body as you exhale.
- Do this process throughout your entire body, paying special attention to the tense and sore areas until you start feeling relaxed in those areas.

Body scan meditation is very important in increasing your body awareness and your ability to recognize when things are going wrong or not working as they should. This type of meditation is a tool that you can use when you are feeling stressed or anxious, and it will help you in releasing tension and becoming more relaxed.

Like in the other types of meditation, our vagus nerve functions best when we are in a relaxed state, so any type of meditation that helps you relax and get into a peaceful state of mind will be instrumental in activating and stimulating your vagus nerve.

Tips For Establishing A Regular Meditation Practice

Establishing a regular meditation practice can have a profound impact on your mental, emotional, and physical well-being. However, starting and maintaining a meditation practice can sometimes be challenging, especially in the beginning. To help you establish a regular meditation practice, here are some tips and strategies to consider:

- **Set Realistic Goals**

Start with realistic goals that are achievable for you. Start with shorter sessions, anywhere from five to ten mins, and slowly work your way up to longer ones as you get more accustomed to the activity. It's better to start small and be consistent rather than aiming for long sessions that you may struggle to maintain.

- **Choose a Convenient Time**

Find a time of the day that works best for you and stick to it. Some people prefer mornings, as it sets a positive tone for the rest of the day, while others find evenings more suitable for relaxation and unwinding. Experiment with different times and determine what fits your schedule and energy levels.

- **Create a Sacred Space**

Designate a specific area in your home as your meditation space. It could be a corner of a room, a cushion, or a small altar. Keep this space clean, clutter-free, and inviting. Adding elements such as candles, incense, or meaningful objects can enhance the ambiance and make it a sacred space for your practice.

- **Start with Guided Meditations**

Guided meditations may serve as a great beginning point for people who are new to meditation or who discover it difficult to sit in silence for long periods of time. There are numerous meditation apps, websites, and YouTube channels that offer guided meditations for various purposes. These guided sessions provide instructions and support, making it easier for beginners to follow along.

- **Experiment with Different Techniques**

There are various meditation techniques available, like mindfulness meditation, loving-kindness meditation, body scan meditation, and transcendental meditation. Experiment with various techniques and find the ones that resonate with you. This variety keeps your practice fresh and allows you to explore different aspects of meditation.

- **Be Gentle with Yourself**

In meditation, it is normal for the mind to move from thought to thought. Once you become aware that your thoughts have wandered off in another direction, return your focus back to the here and now in a calm and collected manner. Avoid judgment or self-criticism. Remember, meditation is a practice, and the mind's tendency to wander is part of the process. Be patient and compassionate with yourself as you cultivate a regular practice.

- **Start with Breathing Exercises**

If sitting in silence feels challenging, begin with simple breathing exercises. Focus on your breath, observing the inhalation and exhalation without judgment. Count your breaths or follow a specific breathing pattern, such as deep belly breathing or box breathing. This helps to calm the mind and establish a foundation for meditation.

- **Use Reminders and Cues**

Place visual reminders or cues around your environment to prompt you to meditate. It could be a sticky note on your mirror, a meditation app notification, or a small object that you associate with your practice. These reminders serve as gentle prompts and encourage you to pause and dedicate time to meditation.

- **Find an Accountability Buddy**

Partnering with someone who shares your interest in meditation can provide accountability and support. You can set meditation goals together, check in on each other's progress, and discuss your experiences. Knowing that someone else is on the same journey can motivate you to maintain consistency.

- **Track Your Progress**

Keep a meditation journal or use a meditation app that allows you to track your practice. Note down the duration of each session, any observations, and how you feel before and after meditation. Tracking your progress not only helps you stay motivated but also allows you to reflect on the benefits and changes that arise from your practice.

- **Be Flexible and Adapt**

Life can be unpredictable, and there may be days when it's challenging to find time for a formal meditation practice. During such times, be flexible and adapt your practice. You can engage in short moments of mindfulness throughout the day, such as mindful breathing during a break or mindful eating during meals. Remember, meditation is not limited to sitting on a cushion—it can be incorporated into various aspects of your daily life.

- **Seek Community and Support**

Consider joining a meditation group or attending meditation retreats or workshops. Being part of a community of like-minded individuals can provide inspiration, guidance, and a sense of belonging. You can learn from experienced practitioners, share your experiences, and deepen your understanding of meditation.

Incorporating Mindfulness Into Daily Activities

The process of paying attention on purpose while reserving judgment on what one sees or experiences in the here and now is the practice of mindfulness. It allows you to fully engage in what you are doing, bringing a greater sense of clarity, peace, and joy to even the simplest of tasks. Listed below are a few suggestions that can help you bring more mindfulness into your daily routine:

Mindful Eating

Instead of rushing through meals or eating on autopilot, take the time to savor and fully experience each bite. Pay attention to the flavors, textures, and smells of your food. Chew slowly and mindfully, noticing the sensation of each bite. Engage your senses and appreciate the nourishment that the food provides.

Mindful Walking

Whether you're taking a stroll in nature or walking from one place to another, use walking as an opportunity for mindfulness. Notice the sensation of your feet touching the ground, the movement of your body, and the surroundings. Pay attention to the sights, sounds, and smells around you. Allow yourself to be fully present in each step.

Mindful Breathing

Throughout the day, take moments to bring your attention to your breath. Direct your attention towards the feeling of your breath as it enters and exits your body. Observe the gentle movement of your belly, noticing how it rises and falls with each breath. Alternatively, you can pay attention to the feeling of air passing through your nostrils, perceiving the coolness during inhalation and the warmth during exhalation. This simple act of mindful breathing can help bring you back to the present moment and create a sense of calm.

Mindful Listening

When engaging in conversations or listening to others, practice active and mindful listening. Give your full attention to the person speaking. Let go of any distractions or the urge to formulate a response in your mind. Instead, truly listen, observing the tone, body language, and emotions behind the words. This deep presence can foster better understanding and connection in your interactions.

Mindful Pause

Incorporate short moments of pause throughout your day. Instead of rushing from one task to another, take a few deep breaths and bring your attention to the present moment. This pause allows you to reset, gather your thoughts, and approach your activities with greater focus and intention.

Mindful Cleaning

Engage in household chores mindfully, turning them into a meditative practice. Whether you're washing dishes, sweeping the floor, or folding laundry, bring your attention fully to the task at hand. Notice the sensations, movements, and sounds involved. Embrace the opportunity to find stillness and clarity in the midst of everyday activities.

Mindful Technology Use

In today's digital age, it's essential to be mindful of our technology use. Set aside dedicated periods of time to disconnect from screens and engage in activities that nourish your mind and body. Practice mindful technology use by being aware of your screen time, setting boundaries, and taking regular breaks to rest and recharge.

Mindful Self-Care

Incorporate mindfulness into your self-care routines. Whether it's taking a relaxing bath, practicing yoga, or enjoying a cup of tea, approach these activities with presence and intention.

Allow yourself to fully immerse in the experience, savoring the sensations and nurturing your well-being.

Mindful Gratitude

Cultivate gratitude by taking a moment each day to reflect on the things you appreciate and are grateful for. It could be as simple as appreciating a beautiful sunrise, a kind gesture from a loved one, or the small joys in your life. Expressing gratitude shifts your focus to the positive aspects of your day and cultivates a mindset of abundance.

Mindful Transitions

Be mindful during transitions between activities. Rather than rushing from one task to another, take a few moments to pause, breathe, and set your intention for the next activity. This helps you to be more present and focused, and it can reduce stress and overwhelm.

Chapter 6:
The Power of Yoga for Vagus Nerve Stimulation

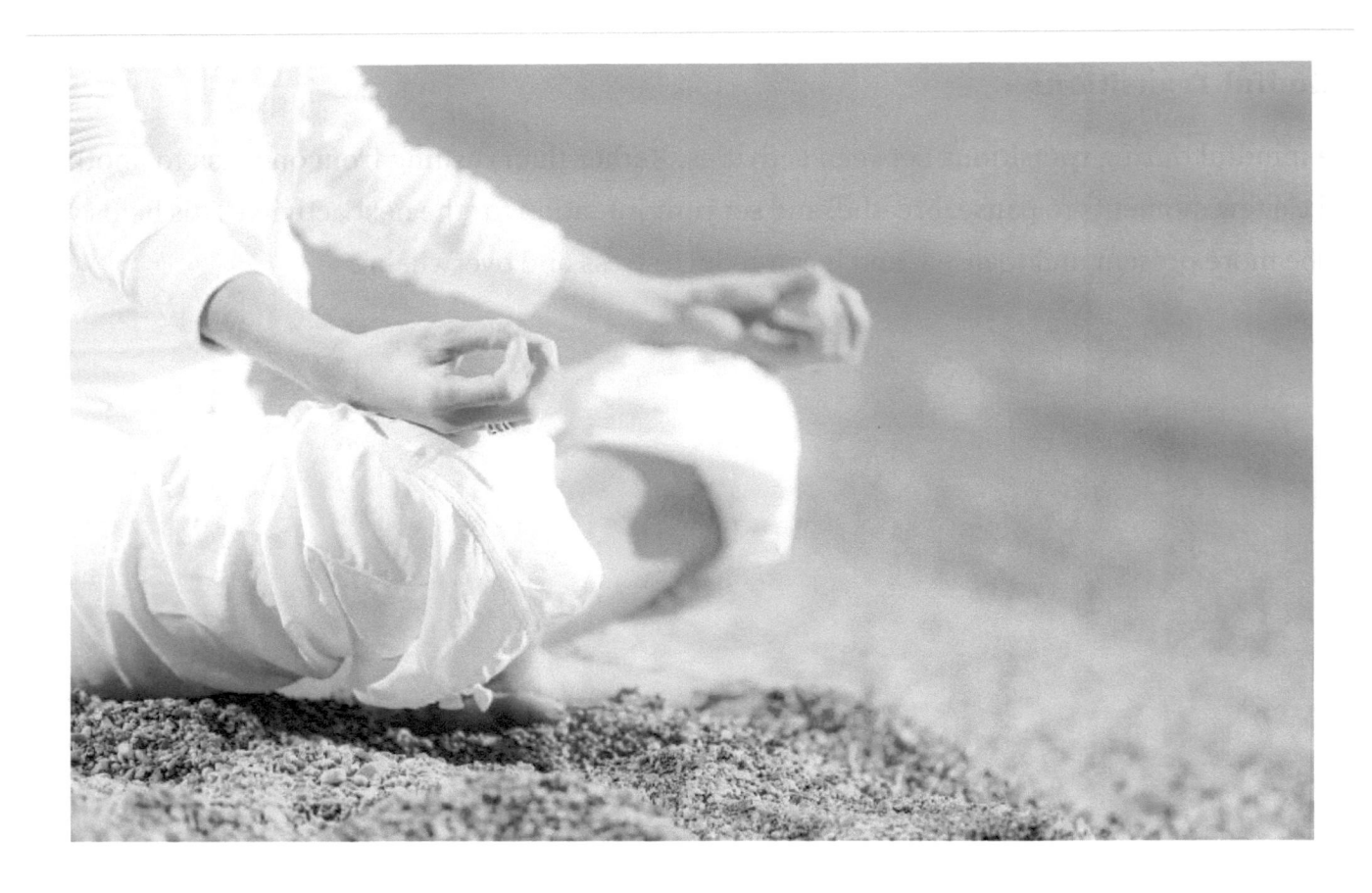

Overview Of Yoga As A Holistic Practice For Mind-Body Wellness

Yoga can be defined as a practice based on harmonizing the mind, body, and soul. By practicing Yoga every day, you will not only explore your true self or your inner self, but also develop the feeling that you are one with nature and environment. Yoga aids the overall well-being of the body and focuses mainly on developing relationship with the natural world around us.

Pain is not just influenced by physical injury or illness, it is also greatly affected by our thoughts, anxiety, trauma, stress and emotions. Stress and pain are closely interrelated - you may experience pain when stressed and stress can also increase the intensity of the pain. When there is increased stress, your breathing becomes heavier, erratic and ragged. Your mood is also altered along with some tension and tightening of the muscles. These symptoms of chronic pain can even increase the toxins in the body and decrease oxygen levels.

Yoga addresses these problems effectively, as it involves the techniques of deep breathing and meditation, which helps in the absorption of much-needed oxygen and also in the relaxation of mind and body. These breathing techniques ensure that the muscles of the lungs, diaphragm, back, and abdomen are fully utilized. When the muscles are loose and relaxed, they can help in releasing the built-up tension in the body and facilitate proper flow of energy throughout. Stress and anxiety levels will also be reduced gradually.

Yoga, or simple stretching, are simple practices that should be applied to everyday life to reduce the tension of stress and keep the muscles in proper working order. There are specific stretches that can focus on problem areas such as the neck or lower back. These stretches can be assigned from a personal trainer, massage therapist, or physiotherapist. Yoga can be enjoyed at home or in a studio with several other participants. There are many forms of yoga ranging from hatha yoga to hot yoga. The focus in yoga is on breath control, meditation, stretching, and balance. Not all forms of yoga are spiritual with chants and mantras, if you don't feel comfortable with that form of practice.

Exercise in general is good for chronic pain, but specific exercises, especially certain yoga positions, help to decrease some types of pain, like shoulder or neck pain.

Additionally, the relaxation techniques you will learn, can teach you how to manage the different types of chronic pain more effectively.

If you are considering trying yoga techniques for your chronic pain, you need to consider the style of yoga you will do.

Specific Yoga Poses And Sequences That Target The Vagus Nerve

In this section, we will delve into a range of yoga poses and sequences specifically designed to target the vagus nerve, fostering its activation and optimal functioning.

1. **Child's Pose (Balasana)**

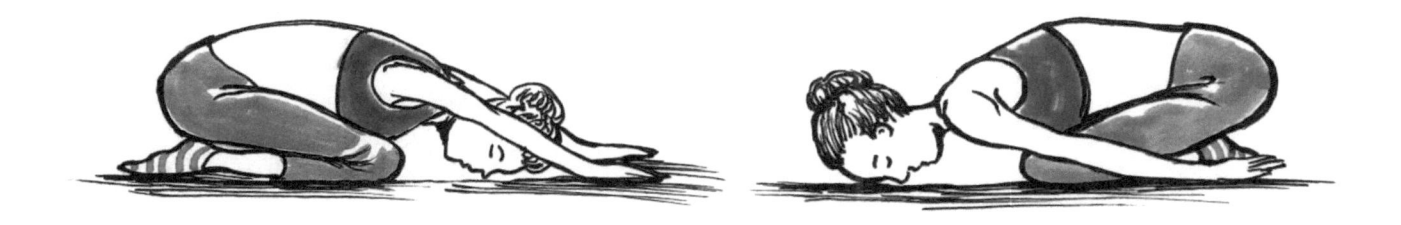

Child's Pose is a gentle and restorative posture that helps to calm the mind, release tension in the body, and stimulate the relaxation response. To practice Child's Pose:

- Begin on your hands and knees, with your knees hip-width apart and your toes touching.
- Begin by sitting back on your heels and gradually lowering your forehead to the mat.
- Extend your arms forward or rest them by your sides, with your palms facing upward.
- Take deep breaths and allow yourself to relax into the posture, enabling your breath to gently massage the area behind your heart and activate the vagus nerve.

Child's Pose fosters a state of relaxation, encourages deep breathing, and promotes a feeling of surrender, all of which contribute to the stimulation of the vagus nerve.

2. Cat-Cow Pose (Marjaryasana-Bitilasana)

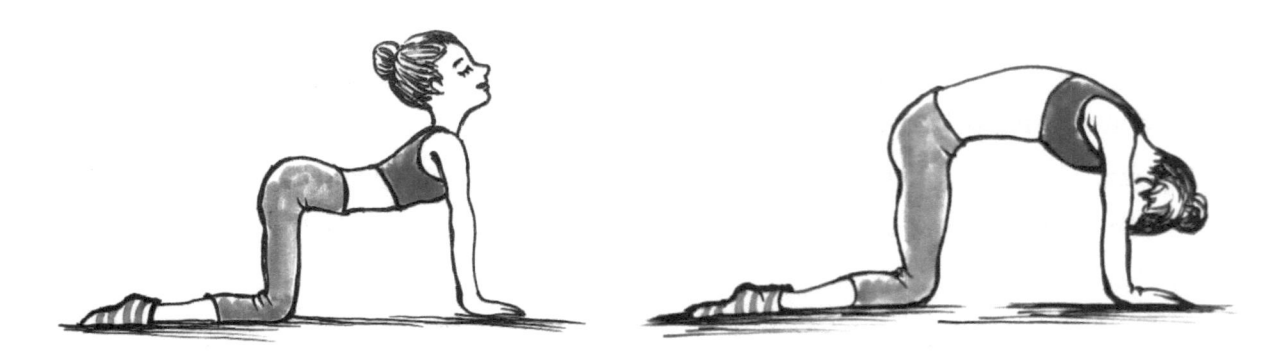

Cat-Cow Pose is a gentle spinal movement that helps to release tension in the spine, open the chest, and promote deep breathing. To practice Cat-Cow Pose:

- Start by positioning yourself on your hands and knees, ensuring that your wrists are directly beneath your shoulders and your knees are aligned with your hips.
- Inhale deeply and lift your chest forward, creating an arch in your back while allowing your belly to sink towards the floor. This is known as the Cow Pose.
- Exhale and round your spine gently, tucking your tailbone under and drawing your belly towards your spine. This is called the Cat Pose.
- Repeat this fluid movement, coordinating each movement with your breath. Cat-Cow Pose promotes the flow of energy in the body, encourages deep diaphragmatic breathing, and activates the vagus nerve.

3. **Legs-Up-The-Wall Pose (Viparita Karani)**

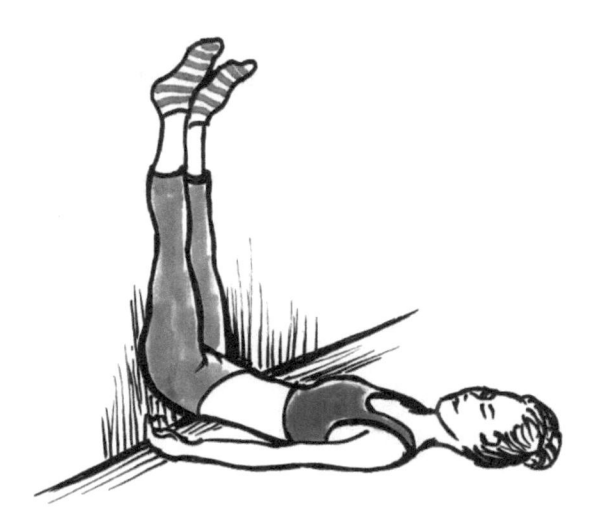

Legs-Up-The-Wall Pose is a gentle inversion that promotes relaxation, soothes the nervous system, and enhances circulation. To practice Legs-Up-The-Wall Pose:

- Sit sideways next to a wall, with your hip touching the wall.
- Lie back and swing your legs up against the wall, keeping your spine straight.
- Relax your arms alongside your body or place them on your belly or chest.
- Close your eyes and focus on your breath, allowing your body to surrender to gravity and the support of the wall. Legs-Up-The-Wall Pose promotes a sense of calm, deep relaxation, and gentle stimulation of the vagus nerve.

4. **Bridge Pose (Setu Bandhasana)**

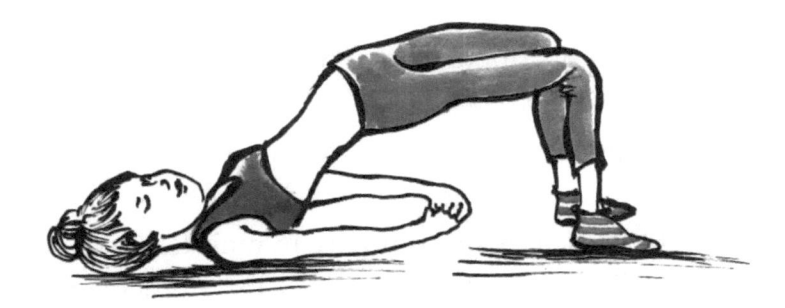

Bridge Pose is a gentle backbend that helps to open the chest, stretch the spine, and stimulate the vagus nerve. To practice Bridge Pose:

- Lie on your back with your knees bent and feet hip-width apart, flat on the floor.
- Press your feet into the floor, engage your glutes, and lift your hips off the mat.
- Interlace your fingers underneath your hips and roll your shoulders back, opening your chest.

- Breathe deeply and hold the pose for several breaths, allowing the breath to reach the back of your throat and stimulate the vagus nerve. Bridge Pose promotes deep breathing, activates the parasympathetic nervous system, and encourages relaxation.

5. **Supported Shoulder Stand (Salamba Sarvangasana)**

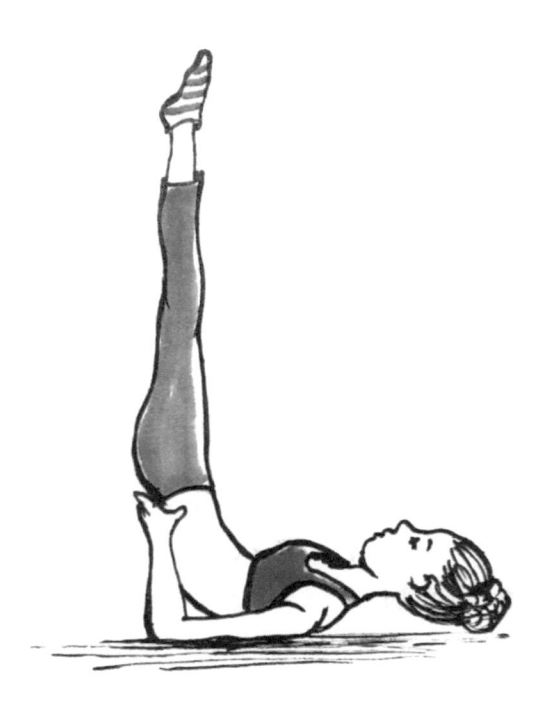

Supported Shoulder Stand is an inversion pose that stimulates the vagus nerve, promotes circulation, and calms the nervous system. To practice Supported Shoulder Stand:

- Lie on your back with your arms alongside your body, palms facing down.
- Lift your legs off the ground, supporting your hips with your hands, and bring your legs perpendicular to the floor.
- Continue to lift your hips and lower back off the mat, supporting your back with your hands.
- Keep your legs straight then activate your core to maintain balance.
- Breathe deeply and hold the pose for several breaths, allowing the gentle pressure on the back of your neck to stimulate the vagus nerve. Supported Shoulder Stand encourages deep breathing, improves circulation, and promotes relaxation.

6. **Corpse Pose (Savasana)**

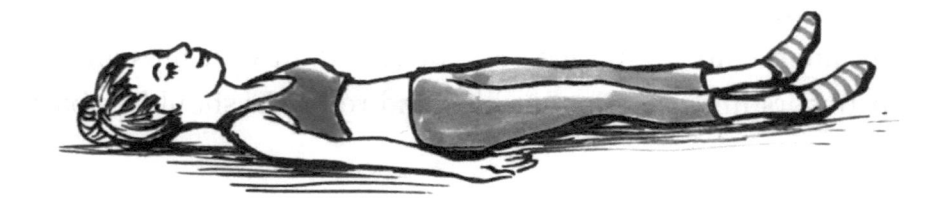

Savasana, also known as Corpse Pose, is a foundational posture in yoga practice. It is typically practiced at the end of a yoga session or as a standalone relaxation pose. Savasana is a time for complete surrender and deep relaxation, allowing the body and mind to integrate the benefits of the practice. To practice Savasana:

- Lie down on your back on a comfortable surface, such as a yoga mat or a soft blanket. Make sure your body is in a straight line, with your legs slightly apart and your arms relaxed by your sides, palms facing up.
- Rest your focus solely on your breathing as you shut your eyes. Begin to deepen and lengthen your inhalations and exhalations, allowing your breath to flow naturally without forcing it.
- Gradually release any tension in your body, starting from your toes and moving all the way up to your head. Consciously relax each part of your body, letting go of any tightness or holding.
- As you settle into the pose, bring your awareness to your breath and the sensations in your body. Notice the gentle rise and fall of your abdomen with each breath. Feel the weight of your body sinking into the ground.
- Let go of any thoughts or mental distractions. If your mind starts to wander, gently bring your focus back to your breath or the physical sensations in your body.
- Remain in Savasana for a few minutes to as long as you like, allowing yourself to completely surrender and experience deep relaxation.

Sequencing these poses together can create a well-rounded practice that targets the vagus nerve and promotes relaxation, deep breathing, and overall well-being. Here's a sample sequence incorporating the poses mentioned above:

1. Begin in Child's Pose for 5-10 breaths, focusing on deep diaphragmatic breathing and relaxation.

2. Move into Cat-Cow Pose, flowing between the two poses for 5-10 rounds of breath, coordinating movement with breath.

3. Transition into Legs-Up-The-Wall Pose and stay for 5-10 minutes, allowing the breath to calm the nervous system and activate the vagus nerve.

4. Release from Legs-Up-The-Wall Pose and come into Bridge Pose for 5-10 breaths, focusing on deep chest and throat breathing.

5. Finish the sequence with Supported Shoulder Stand, holding the pose for 5-10 breaths, and allowing the gentle inversion to stimulate the vagus nerve.

6. After completing the poses, take a few minutes in Savasana (Corpse Pose) to integrate the effects of the practice and observe any changes in your body and mind.

Remember to approach your yoga practice with mindfulness, honoring your body's needs and limitations. As you practice these poses and sequences, listen to your body, breathe deeply, and allow the practices to support the activation and stimulation of your vagus nerve, promoting relaxation, well-being, and balance in your life.

Incorporating Breathwork And Movement In Yoga For Vagus Nerve Activation

Incorporating breathwork and movement in yoga can be a powerful way to activate and stimulate the vagus nerve. By intentionally combining specific breathwork techniques and movement in yoga, we can enhance vagal tone and experience the many benefits associated with vagus nerve activation. Here's how you can incorporate breathwork and movement in yoga for vagus nerve activation:

1. **Deep Belly Breathing (Diaphragmatic Breathing)**

Deep belly breathing is a foundational breathwork technique that helps activate the relaxation response and stimulate the vagus nerve. To begin, locate a position that feels comfortable for you, whether it's seated or lying down. Place one hand on your belly and the other on your chest. As you breathe, focus on taking slow and deep breaths. Allow your belly to naturally rise with each inhalation and fall with each exhalation. Focus on expanding your diaphragm and fully engaging your breath in the lower belly. Practice this breathwork technique at the start and end of your yoga session to promote relaxation and activate the vagus nerve.

2. **Ujjayi Breath (Victorious Breath)**

Ujjayi breath is a breathing technique commonly used in yoga to cultivate internal heat and focus the mind. A mild, audible sound is produced by inhaling and exhaling via the nose whilst gently contracting the back of the throat. This is done when doing the nasal breathing technique. This intentional breath control stimulates the vagus nerve and promotes a sense of calm and centeredness. Incorporate Ujjayi breath throughout your yoga practice, especially during more challenging poses or sequences, to enhance vagal tone and deepen your mind-body connection.

3. **Gentle Backbends**

Backbending poses in yoga, such as Cobra Pose (Bhujangasana) or Bridge Pose (Setu Bandhasana), can help stimulate the vagus nerve. These gentle backbends open the front body, expand the chest, and create space in the throat and neck region where the vagus nerve resides.

Practice these poses mindfully, focusing on deep breaths and creating length and extension in the spine. Remember to listen to your body and adjust the poses as needed.

4. Supported Inversion

Inversions, where the head is below the heart, are known to have a calming effect on the nervous system and activate the vagus nerve. Supported inversions like Legs-Up-The-Wall Pose (Viparita Karani) or Supported Shoulder Stand (Salamba Sarvangasana) are accessible options that promote relaxation and enhance vagal tone. These poses increase blood flow to the brain and stimulate the vagus nerve through gentle pressure on the back of the neck. Practice these poses with the support of props and guidance from an experienced yoga teacher.

5. Gentle Twists

Twisting poses in yoga, such as Seated Spinal Twist (Ardha Matsyendrasana) or Supine Twist (Supta Matsyendrasana), can help massage the abdominal organs and stimulate the vagus nerve. Twists promote digestion, release tension in the abdomen, and increase circulation in the torso. As you twist, focus on maintaining a long spine and incorporating deep, steady breaths to maximize the benefits of vagus nerve activation.

6. Restorative Yoga

Restorative yoga is a gentle and nurturing practice that emphasizes deep relaxation and rejuvenation. It involves the use of props to support the body in passive poses for extended periods. Restorative poses like Supported Child's Pose (Balasana), Supported Heart Opener (Supported Fish Pose), or Legs-Up-The-Wall Pose provide a sense of grounding, calm, and deep rest. By allowing the body to fully relax and surrender, we create an ideal environment for vagus nerve activation and the release of tension and stress.

7. Mindful Savasana (Corpse Pose)

Savasana is the final relaxation pose in yoga, often referred to as Corpse Pose. It is a time for complete surrender and integration of the practice. As you lie flat on your back, bring your awareness to your breath, allowing it to become slow and steady. Scan your body for any areas of tension and consciously release them. Visualize a sense of softness and relaxation spreading throughout your entire being. By practicing mindful Savasana, you give the vagus nerve a chance to recalibrate the nervous system and promote deep relaxation and restoration.

Chapter 7:
Engaging the Senses: Sound and Vagus Nerve Stimulation

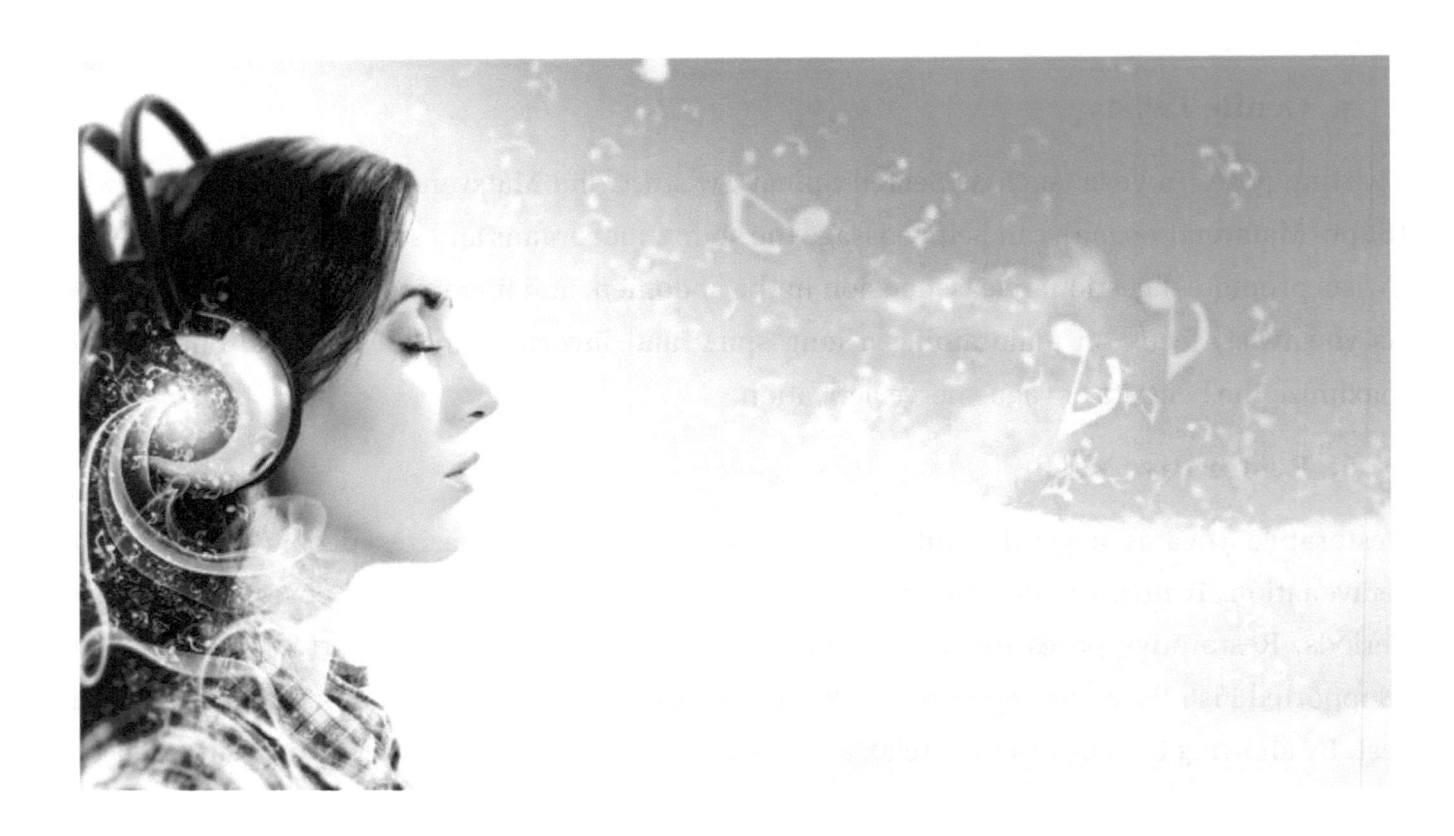

The Therapeutic Effects Of Sound On The Vagus Nerve

Sound therapy, specifically through techniques such as music, chanting, singing bowls, and certain frequencies, has been found to have therapeutic effects on the vagus nerve. The vagus nerve is intricately connected to the auditory system, and various studies have shown that specific sounds can stimulate and activate the vagus nerve, leading to several beneficial outcomes. Here are the therapeutic effects of sound on the vagus nerve:

- Vagal Tone Enhancement: Vagal tone refers to the activity level of the vagus nerve. Higher vagal tone is associated with better overall health, emotional regulation, and stress resilience. Sound therapy, especially through calming and soothing sounds, has been shown to enhance vagal tone. Listening to gentle and harmonious music or chanting can promote relaxation, reduce stress, and improve vagal tone, leading to increased well-being.

- Stress Reduction and Relaxation: Sound therapy has a direct impact on the body's stress response, activating the parasympathetic nervous system and promoting relaxation. By listening to calming sounds or specific frequencies, such as binaural beats, the vagus nerve can be stimulated, triggering the release of neurotransmitters that induce relaxation and counteract the effects of stress.
- Heart Rate Variability (HRV) Improvement: Heart rate variability is the variation in the time interval between heartbeats and is an indicator of autonomic nervous system balance. Increased HRV, particularly in the high-frequency range, is associated with better overall health and vagal nerve activity. Sound therapy, such as listening to certain types of music, has been shown to improve HRV by enhancing vagal nerve function and promoting a more balanced autonomic nervous system.
- Emotional Regulation and Mood Enhancement: Sound therapy can have a profound impact on emotional well-being and mood regulation. Listening to uplifting and soothing sounds can positively affect neurotransmitter release, including dopamine and serotonin, which are involved in mood regulation. As the vagus nerve is connected to brain regions involved in emotional processing, sound therapy can stimulate the vagus nerve, promoting emotional regulation, reducing symptoms of anxiety and depression, and enhancing overall mood.
- Enhanced Mind-Body Connection: Sound therapy can facilitate a deeper connection between the mind and body. By engaging with specific sounds or vibrations, individuals can cultivate a heightened sense of body awareness and promote a state of relaxation and inner harmony. This connection between sound and the vagus nerve can foster a greater sense of well-being and balance in both physical and emotional aspects.
- Improved Sleep Quality: Sound therapy can positively impact sleep quality by promoting relaxation and reducing factors that disrupt sleep, such as stress and anxiety. Listening to calming sounds, nature sounds, or white noise can create a soothing environment that encourages deep sleep and relaxation. As the vagus nerve is involved in the regulation of sleep and wakefulness, sound therapy can indirectly support better sleep patterns.
- Pain Management: Sound therapy has been explored as a complementary approach for pain management. By engaging with specific sounds or frequencies, individuals may experience a reduction in pain perception and increased pain tolerance. The vagus nerve's activation through sound therapy can modulate pain pathways and trigger the release of endogenous opioids, which have analgesic effects.

Using Music And Sound Therapy For Relaxation And Stress Reduction

Music and sound therapy are effective techniques for relaxation and stress reduction. The rhythmic patterns, melodies, and vibrations of music can have a profound impact on our physiology, emotions, and overall well-being. Here's how you can use music and sound therapy to promote relaxation and reduce stress:

Select Calming Music

Choose music that has a soothing and calming effect on you. This can vary depending on personal preferences, but genres like classical, ambient, instrumental, or nature sounds tend to be popular choices. Experiment with different styles to find what resonates with you and evokes a sense of relaxation.

Create a Relaxing Environment

Set the stage for relaxation by creating a peaceful and comfortable environment. Find a quiet space where you can listen to music without distractions. Dim the lights, light some candles, or use essential oils to enhance the sensory experience and create a calming ambiance.

Deep Breathing and Mindful Listening

Sit or lie down in a comfortable position and focus on your breath. Take slow, deep breaths, allowing your body to relax with each exhale. As you listen to the music, direct your attention to the sounds, melodies, and rhythms. Engage in mindful listening, fully immersing yourself in the music and letting go of any racing thoughts or worries.

Progressive Muscle Relaxation

Combine music therapy with progressive muscle relaxation techniques. While you are listening to the music, carefully contract and relax every muscle group in your body, beginning with your toes then progressing your way towards your head. This combination of music and muscle relaxation can amplify the relaxation response and release tension from your body.

Guided Imagery

Use music as a backdrop for guided imagery exercises. Close your eyes and imagine yourself in a peaceful and serene place, like a beach, forest, or meadow. Visualize the details, sounds, and sensations of this imaginary place while allowing the music to enhance the experience. This combination of music and guided imagery can transport you to a state of deep relaxation.

Singing or Chanting

Engage in singing or chanting practices to promote relaxation and stress reduction. Singing or chanting repetitive mantras or soothing melodies can have a calming effect on the nervous system. It helps regulate your breathing, activates the vagus nerve, and releases endorphins, promoting a sense of well-being and stress relief.

Use Sound Healing Instruments

Explore the use of sound healing instruments like singing bowls, gongs, or tuning forks. These instruments produce resonant and harmonious sounds that can induce a meditative state, reduce stress, and promote relaxation. Allow the sounds to wash over you, focusing on the vibrations and their soothing effects.

Incorporate Music into Daily Activities

Integrate relaxing music into your daily activities to create a calming atmosphere. Listen to calming playlists during your morning routine, while commuting, or before bed. This can help counteract stressors and create a more tranquil environment throughout your day.

Guided Auditory Exercises For Vagus Nerve Activation

Guided auditory exercises can be a powerful tool for activating and stimulating the vagus nerve. These exercises use specific sounds, tones, and frequencies to target the vagus nerve, promoting relaxation, stress reduction, and overall well-being. Here are some guided auditory exercises that you can incorporate into your routine:

1. **Binaural Beats**

Binaural beats involve playing two slightly different frequencies in each ear, creating a perceived third frequency in the brain. This technique can help synchronize brainwaves and induce a state of relaxation. To experience the benefits of binaural beats for vagus nerve activation, follow these steps:

- Find a comfortable and quiet space.
- Wear headphones to ensure each ear receives a separate frequency.
- Choose a binaural beats track that is designed for relaxation and vagus nerve activation.
- Close your eyes, relax your body, and focus on the sounds.
- Allow the binaural beats to guide your brainwaves into a more relaxed state, promoting vagus nerve stimulation.

2. Humming and Chanting

Humming and chanting produce specific vibrations and frequencies that can stimulate the vagus nerve. The vibrations created by vocalizing these sounds can help activate the relaxation response and enhance vagal tone. Here's how to incorporate humming and chanting into your vagus nerve activation practice:

- Find a quiet and comfortable space.
- Sit in a relaxed position and take a few deep breaths to center yourself.
- Start humming softly, focusing on the vibration in your throat and chest.
- Gradually increase the volume and intensity of your hum, feeling the vibrations resonating throughout your body.
- Alternatively, you can chant specific sounds or mantras, such as "OM" or "Ah," and feel the resonance in your body as you repeat the sounds.

3. Resonant Breathing

Resonant breathing, also known as coherent breathing, is a technique that involves matching your breath with a specific rhythm to promote relaxation and vagal nerve stimulation. Here's how to practice resonant breathing:

- Locate a spot that is serene, cozy, and suitable for sitting or lying down.
- For a moment of relaxation, try closing your eyes and taking some deep breaths for a couple of moments.
- Take four slow, deliberate, and deep breaths via your nose while counting to four.
- Blow out an air breath via your nose, counting to four as you do it slowly and fully.
- Continue this breathing pattern, maintaining a smooth and rhythmic flow of breath.
- As you breathe, focus your attention on the sensations of your breath, allowing it to create a calming and relaxing effect throughout your body.

4. Singing Bowls

Singing bowls produce resonant sounds that can help activate the vagus nerve and induce a state of relaxation. Here's how to use singing bowls for vagus nerve activation:

- Find a quiet and comfortable space.
- Place the singing bowl in front of you, ensuring it is secure on a cushion or mat.
- Gently strike the bowl or use a rubbing technique to create a sustained sound.
- As the sound begins to resonate, focus your attention on the vibrations and allow them to penetrate your body.

- Continue to listen to the sound and feel the vibrations as they promote relaxation and vagus nerve stimulation.

5. Nature Sounds

Nature sounds, such as ocean waves, rain, or birdsong, have a calming effect on the nervous system and can help activate the vagus nerve. Here's how to incorporate nature sounds into your vagus nerve activation practice:

- Find a comfortable and quiet space.
- Play a recording of nature sounds or use a nature sound app.
- Close your eyes and listen to the sounds.
- Visualize yourself in a natural setting, immersing yourself in the sounds and sensations of nature.
- Allow the soothing sounds to promote relaxation and stimulate the vagus nerve.

6. Guided Imagery

Guided imagery combines soothing auditory cues with visualization to promote relaxation and vagal nerve activation. Here's how to practice guided imagery for vagus nerve stimulation:

- Find a quiet and comfortable space.
- Close your eyes and take a few deep breaths to relax.
- Listen to a guided imagery recording that incorporates relaxing sounds and visualizations.
- Follow the instructions provided, allowing your mind to create vivid images and sensations that promote relaxation and vagal nerve stimulation.

These guided auditory exercises can be practiced individually or in combination, depending on your preferences and needs. Experiment with various techniques and explore what works best for you. By incorporating these exercises into your routine, you can tap into the power of sound and vibration to activate and stimulate the vagus nerve, promoting relaxation, stress reduction, and overall well-being.

Chapter 8:

Physical Exercises and Bodywork

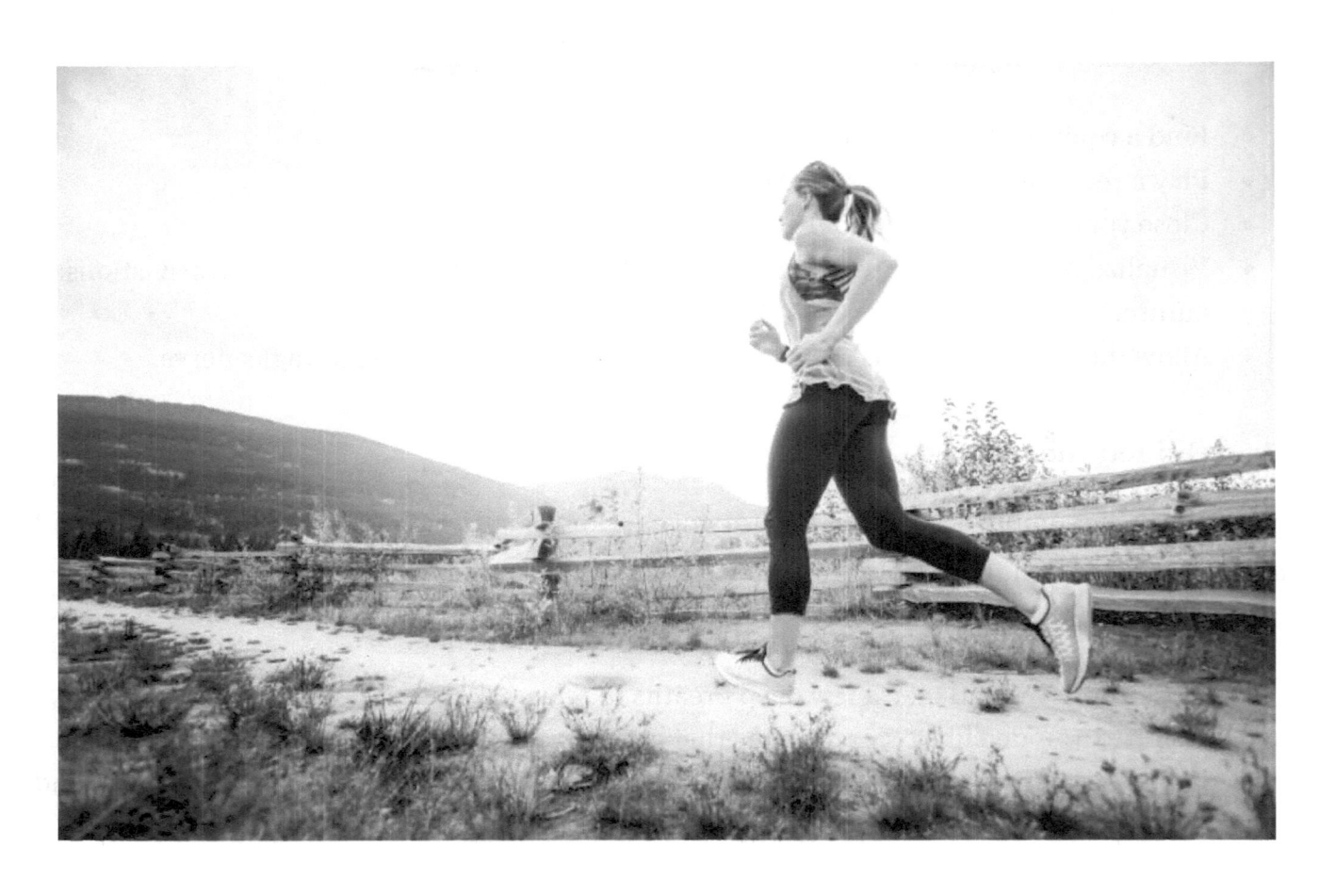

Understanding The Link Between Physical Activity And Vagus Nerve Function

Regular physical activity, especially aerobic exercise, has been found to have a positive influence on the function of the vagus nerve. Consistent exercise stimulates the vagus nerve, resulting in an enhancement of vagal tone. A higher vagal tone is associated with many health benefits, comprising enhanced cardiovascular health, better emotional regulation, elevated stress resilience, and overall well-being.

During exercise, the body experiences an increase in heart rate and respiration rate, which activates the sympathetic nervous system, preparing the body for action. However, it is the parasympathetic nervous system, governed by the vagus nerve, that promotes relaxation and facilitates recovery after physical exertion. Engaging in aerobic activities like jogging, swimming, or cycling specifically activates the parasympathetic branch of the autonomic nervous system, resulting in an elevation of vagal activity and a shift towards a more relaxed state.

Higher vagal tone induced by physical activity has several benefits. It helps regulate heart rate and blood pressure, promotes efficient digestion, enhances immune system function, and supports emotional well-being.

In addition to these specific benefits, physical activity also promotes overall well-being by improving sleep quality, enhancing cognitive function and neuroplasticity, and reducing the risk of chronic diseases such as obesity, diabetes, and certain cancers. The vagus nerve, through its influence on various physiological systems, contributes to these positive outcomes.

Cardiovascular Exercises For Vagus Nerve Stimulation

Cardiovascular exercises increase heart rate, respiration, and oxygen consumption, leading to a cascade of physiological effects that activate the parasympathetic nervous system, regulated by the vagus nerve. Here are some cardiovascular exercises that can help stimulate the vagus nerve:

1. **Aerobic Exercises**

Running or Jogging: Running or jogging at a moderate to high intensity can effectively stimulate the vagus nerve. Start with a warm-up, then maintain a steady pace for a duration of time that challenges you.

Cycling: Whether indoors on a stationary bike or outdoors on a bicycle, cycling is a great cardiovascular exercise that can stimulate the vagus nerve. Adjust the intensity and duration based on your fitness level.

Swimming: Swimming is a low-impact, full-body workout that can provide a stimulating effect on the vagus nerve. Aim for sustained periods of swimming at a moderate intensity.

2. **High-Intensity Interval Training (HIIT)**

HIIT involves alternating periods of high-intensity exercise with short recovery periods. This type of workout can be effective in stimulating the vagus nerve due to its combination of intense effort followed by brief rest. Examples include sprint intervals, burpees, or jumping jacks.

3. **Dance Aerobics**

Dance-based aerobic workouts, such as Zumba or dance cardio classes, can be enjoyable ways to stimulate the vagus nerve. The combination of rhythmic movements, music, and elevated heart rate can promote vagal activation and overall well-being.

4. Jumping Rope

Jumping rope is a simple yet effective cardiovascular exercise that can be done almost anywhere. It involves repetitive movements that elevate heart rate and engage multiple muscle groups, providing a vagus nerve-stimulating effect.

5. Elliptical Training

Using an elliptical machine provides a low-impact cardiovascular workout that can effectively stimulate the vagus nerve. Adjust the resistance and incline to vary the intensity and challenge your cardiovascular system.

6. Kickboxing

Kickboxing workouts combine cardiovascular exercise with martial arts movements. The high-intensity nature of kickboxing can stimulate the vagus nerve while providing a full-body workout.

When engaging in cardiovascular exercises for vagus nerve stimulation, it is essential to pay attention to what your body is telling you and to begin at a level which is suitable for your current level of fitness. Slowly elevate the intensity and duration over time as you build endurance and strength. It's also essential to warm up before each exercise session and cool down afterward to prevent injury and promote recovery.

Remember to pay attention to your breathing during cardiovascular exercises. Slow, deep breaths can enhance vagal activation and further stimulate the relaxation response. Focusing on diaphragmatic breathing, where you breathe deeply into your abdomen, can help maximize the benefits of vagus nerve stimulation during exercise.

Incorporating cardiovascular exercises into your regular routine can not only improve cardiovascular fitness but also provide a natural and effective way to stimulate the vagus nerve. By promoting vagal activation, these exercises contribute to stress reduction, emotional well-being, improved digestion, and overall health.

Massage Techniques For Vagus Nerve Activation And Relaxation

Massage techniques can be effective in activating the vagus nerve and promoting relaxation. By incorporating specific massage techniques, you can stimulate the vagus nerve and induce a relaxation response in the body. Here are some massage techniques that can help activate the vagus nerve and promote relaxation:

1. **Neck and Throat Massage**

- Gently massage the sides of your neck using circular motions with your fingertips or the palms of your hands. Start from the base of your skull and move down towards your shoulders. Apply gentle pressure and focus on any areas of tension.
- Massage the front of your throat using light, upward strokes. Be gentle and avoid putting too much pressure on the sensitive structures in the neck.

2. **Ear Massage**

- Gently rub your earlobes between your thumb and index finger. Move your fingers in circular motions, gradually working your way up the outer edges of your ears.
- Use your fingertips to apply gentle pressure to the area just behind your ears, where the mastoid bone is located. Apply circular motions or small vibrations to this area.

3. **Abdominal Massage**

- Lie down in a comfortable position and place your hands on your abdomen.
- Using gentle circular motions, massage your abdomen in a clockwise direction. Start from the lower right side and move upward, then across to the left side and downward.
- Apply light pressure and focus on relaxation rather than deep tissue manipulation.

4. **Face Massage**

- Begin by placing your fingertips on your temples and apply gentle circular motions.
- Move your fingertips down to your cheeks and massage in upward strokes towards your temples.
- Use your fingertips to massage the area around your jaw joints in circular motions.

5. **Foot Massage**

- Sit down and place one foot on the opposite thigh, exposing the sole of your foot.
- Use your hands, thumbs, or a massage tool to apply pressure and massage the sole of your foot. Start from the heel and move towards the toes, focusing on the arch and the ball of the foot.
- Repeat the process on the other foot.

6. Self-Compassion Touch

- Place your hands on your chest, one hand over the other, with your fingertips resting lightly on your collarbones.
- Close your eyes, take a deep breath, and allow your body to relax.
- Apply gentle pressure with your hands and focus on the sensations of touch and warmth. Practice self-compassion and send kind thoughts to yourself.

When practicing these massage techniques, it's important to create a calm and soothing environment. Use relaxing music, dim lighting, and scented candles or essential oils to enhance the relaxation experience. Take slow, deep breaths during the massage to further promote relaxation and activate the vagus nerve.

The vagus nerve is closely connected to the face, neck, throat, abdomen, and ears, making these areas particularly effective for vagus nerve activation. By applying gentle pressure and using circular motions, these massage techniques stimulate the nerve endings and sensory receptors in these regions, which in turn activate the vagus nerve.

Massage not only activates the vagus nerve but also promotes the release of endorphins and reduces the levels of stress hormones such as cortisol. This leads to a decrease in sympathetic nervous system activity and an increase in parasympathetic activity, resulting in a state of relaxation and calmness.

Chapter 9:
Lifestyle and Self-Care Practices for Vagus Nerve Health

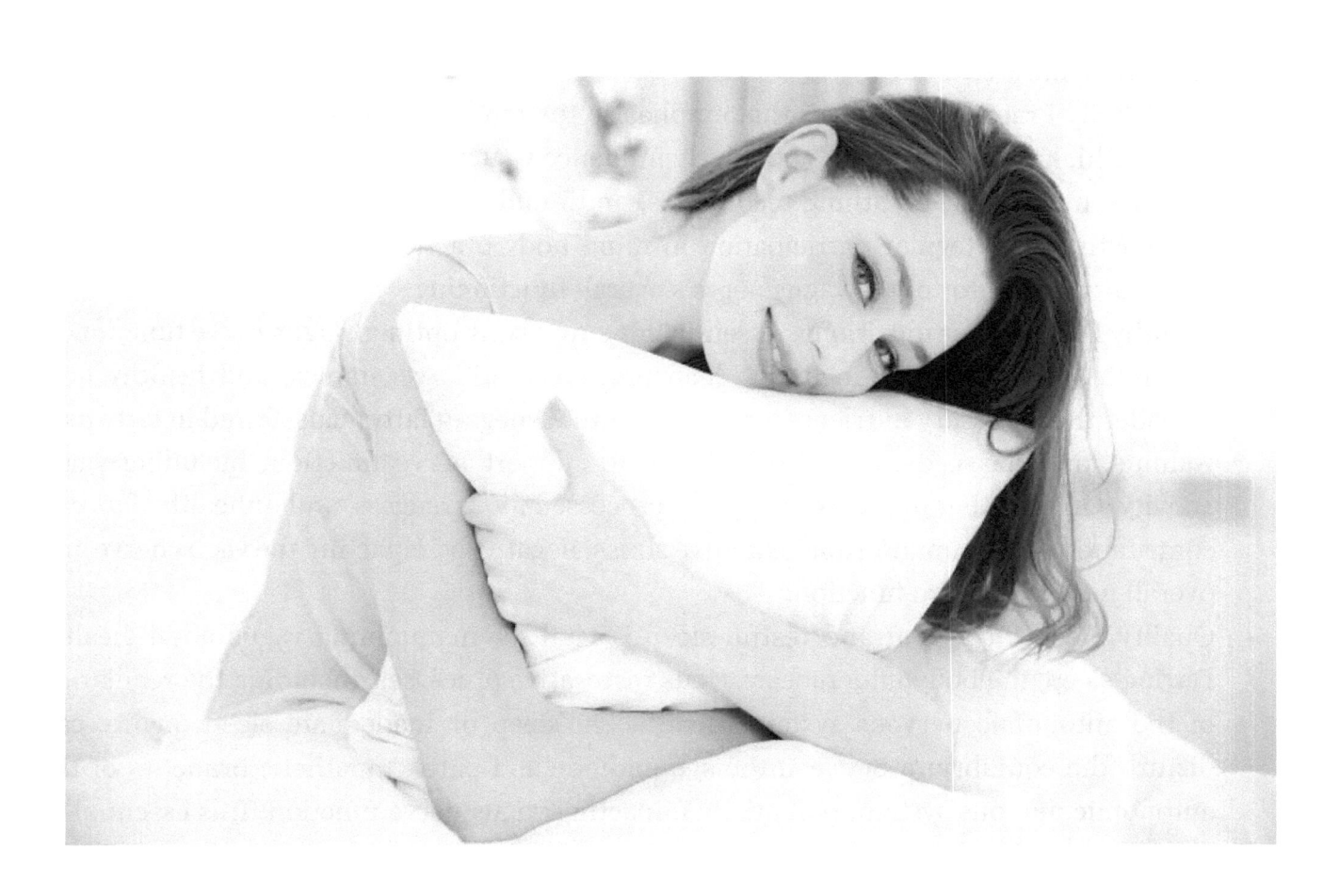

Importance Of A Healthy Lifestyle In Supporting Vagus Nerve Function

A healthy lifestyle is crucial for supporting optimal vagus nerve function. The vagus nerve plays a fundamental role in regulating various physiological processes in the body. By adopting healthy lifestyle habits, we can positively impact the vagus nerve and promote overall well-being. Here are some reasons why a healthy lifestyle is important for supporting vagus nerve function:

- Stress Reduction: Chronic stress negatively impacts vagus nerve function, leading to a dysregulated stress response and increased sympathetic nervous system activity.

Adopting stress management techniques such as regular exercise, mindfulness meditation, and adequate sleep can help reduce stress levels and enhance vagus nerve activity. These practices promote a shift towards a more relaxed state, activating the parasympathetic branch of the autonomic nervous system, which is regulated by the vagus nerve.

- Regular Physical Activity: Engaging in regular physical activity is not only beneficial for cardiovascular health but also promotes vagus nerve stimulation. Aerobic exercises, such as swimming, jogging, or cycling, increase heart rate, respiration, and oxygen consumption, leading to an activation of the parasympathetic nervous system. This activation stimulates the vagus nerve, enhancing its function and promoting overall relaxation and well-being.
- Mind-Body Practices: Practices that emphasize the mind-body connection, such as yoga and tai chi, have been found to positively influence vagus nerve function. These practices combine movement, breathing techniques, and mindfulness, promoting relaxation and vagal activation. Regular participation in mind-body practices can improve vagal tone, which is an indicator of the vagus nerve's overall functioning.
- Healthy Diet: Proper nutrition is essential for supporting optimal vagus nerve function. A diet rich in whole foods, including lean proteins, fruits, vegetables, and healthy fats, provides the necessary nutrients for nerve health. Omega-3 fatty acids, found in fatty fish, walnuts, and flaxseeds, have been shown to support nerve function, including vagal activity. On the other hand, a diet high in processed foods, sugars, and unhealthy fats can contribute to inflammation and oxidative stress, negatively impacting the vagus nerve and overall nervous system function.
- Quality Sleep: Sufficient and restful sleep is vital for maintaining vagus nerve health. During sleep, the body undergoes various restorative processes, including the regulation of the autonomic nervous system. Insufficient sleep or inadequate sleep quality can disturb the equilibrium between the sympathetic and parasympathetic branches of the autonomic nervous system, potentially impacting vagus nerve function. It is essential to establish healthy sleep practices to promote optimal vagal activity and enhance overall well-being.
- Emotional Well-being: Emotional well-being is closely tied to vagus nerve function. Practices that promote emotional resilience, such as practicing gratitude, cultivating positive relationships, and engaging in activities that bring joy, positively influence the vagus nerve. Chronic negative emotions, such as anxiety, depression, and chronic stress, can impair vagal function. By prioritizing emotional well-being and seeking support when needed, we can support vagus nerve health and enhance our ability to manage stress and regulate emotions.
- Social Connection: Human connection and social support have been linked to improved vagus nerve function. Engaging in meaningful relationships, connecting with loved ones, and participating in community activities promote a sense of belonging and emotional

well-being, which positively influence vagal tone. Regular social interaction and the cultivation of positive social bonds contribute to a healthy vagus nerve and overall nervous system function.

These lifestyle factors contribute to a balanced autonomic nervous system, promoting a state of relaxation, resilience, and overall well-being. Nurturing the vagus nerve through a healthy lifestyle is an investment in our long-term health and can positively impact various aspects of our physical, mental, and emotional health.

Nutrition Tips For Optimal Vagus Nerve Health

Proper nutrition is essential for maintaining optimal health of the vagus nerve. As previously discussed, the vagus nerve is involved in numerous bodily functions, such as digestion, inflammation regulation, mood control, and immune response. By embracing a well-rounded and nutrient-rich diet, we can supply the vital nutrients needed to support the function of the vagus nerve and promote overall well-being. Consider the following nutrition tips to enhance the health of your vagus nerve:

1. **Omega-3 Fatty Acids**

Fatty fish, such as sardines, mackerel and salmon are excellent sources of omega-3 fatty acids. These fish contain high levels of docosahexaenoic acid (DHA) and eicosapentaenoic acid (EPA), two types of omega-3s that are particularly beneficial for nerve health. Consuming fatty fish regularly can supply your body with a significant amount of omega-3s, which can support the functioning of the vagus nerve.

2. **Antioxidant-Rich Foods**

Oxidative stress can have detrimental effects on nerve health, including the vagus nerve. Including anti-oxidant rich foods in your diet can help counteract oxidative stress and support optimal nerve function. Antioxidant-rich foods include a variety of options such as berries (raspberries, blueberries, strawberries), leafy green vegetables (spinach, kale), colorful fruits and vegetables (oranges, carrots, bell peppers), as well as nuts and seeds.

3. **B Vitamins**

B vitamins are crucial for nerve health and function, including the vagus nerve. They play a role in the production and maintenance of myelin, a protective sheath around nerve cells. Good sources of B vitamins include whole grains, legumes, leafy green vegetables, eggs, dairy products, lean meats, and seafood.

4. Magnesium

Magnesium is an essential mineral that supports nerve function, including the vagus nerve. It helps regulate neurotransmitter activity and promotes relaxation. Excellent dietary sources of magnesium comprise leafy green vegetables, nuts and seeds (such as almonds, cashews, and pumpkin seeds), legumes, whole grains, and dark chocolate. Including magnesium-rich foods in your diet can support vagus nerve health and overall relaxation.

5. Probiotic-Rich Foods

The gut-brain connection is closely linked to vagus nerve function. Consuming probiotic-rich foods can support a healthy gut microbiome, which in turn positively influences vagus nerve activity. Fermented foods like yogurt, kefir, sauerkraut, kimchi, and kombucha are excellent sources of probiotics. Including these foods in your diet can promote gut health and vagus nerve function.

6. Healthy Fats

Including healthy fats in your diet is essential for nerve health, as nerve cells rely on fats for proper functioning. Healthy fats, like those found in olive oil, avocados, coconut oil, nuts, and seeds, provide a source of energy and support the integrity of nerve cell membranes. Including these in your diet can support vagus nerve health and overall nerve function.

7. Avoiding Inflammatory Foods

Chronic inflammation can negatively impact vagus nerve function. To support optimal vagus nerve health, it's important to minimize the consumption of inflammatory foods. These include highly processed and refined foods, sugary snacks and beverages, excessive amounts of saturated and trans fats, and foods high in additives and preservatives. Instead, focus on whole, unprocessed foods that are rich in nutrients.

8. Adequate Hydration

Staying hydrated is essential for overall health, including nerve function. Dehydration can affect nerve transmission and impair vagus nerve activity. Aim to drink an adequate amount of water throughout the day to maintain hydration and support optimal nerve function.

Quality Sleep And Its Impact On The Vagus Nerve

Sleep - all of us need it, so you may not rest as much as you want as you have extreme depression or an anxiety disorder. You may have trouble eating or exercising, partially because you don't have to escape from your restless mind and body when you relax and turn the lights off. This is when worries and anxieties move in, which makes the night turn and jump. You can guarantee you're in for a tough night if you then start to be worried that you don't sleep or not sleep well.

Roughly 30% of adults suffer at some point in their life with sleeplessness (difficulty sleeping). When you are women or an older adult, your risk of sleeplessness is higher, and when mening and menopause start, you have a higher risk of sleeplessness in women. About 40% of insomnia patients have depression and mood disorder. You probably noticed that you feel more anxious and worried during the day as you sleep in poor condition. This pattern of depression, sleep deprivation, stress, and sleep is a dangerous process in many people with anxiety problems.

Many people get 7 to 8 hours per night of sleep, and people get the most from almost 6 hrs of sleep per night. The body knows the way it wants to sleep and, in the early hours of the night, it becomes the longest and most essential sleep so that you can function properly. Nevertheless, the quantity and quality of your sleep could be influenced by different medical conditions. If you snore, have sleeping trouble or experience leg cramps or tingling (possible sleep apnea symptoms), have gastrointestinal discomfort, regular leg movements and chronic nightly pain that stops you from sleeping easily, talk to your doctor or a specialist for sleep.

Tips for a Better Night's Sleep

Several things can make a good night's sleep complicated for you. Many causes, such as too much caffeine or too late in the day, maybe noticeable. The quantity and quality of your sleep can affect your sleep habits too. Here are some sleep expert tips to help you get to sleep more effectively in the night.

Allow sleep to come naturally. When you are ready, you do not "go to sleep." In other words, you can't control sleep and you can't go to bed, regardless of how hard you try. Sleep automatically takes place, and the best you can do is leave. If you're afraid to sleep, it could be very tough for you to get out of the house. However, if you're ready it's the most beneficial attitude to be resting. So, what are you doing while you are waiting to sleep? Don't fight it if you can't fall asleep in 30 minutes. Get out of bed and try some relaxing tasks like yoga, reading, knitting, and painting. Go back to bed if you start to feel drowsy. Seek to do the same thing again if you're already sleeping in another 30 minutes. Nonetheless, don't make it to get sleep to come because of what you do while waiting for sleep to arrive.

Don't nap or catch up on weekends. Sleep pressure is that feeling of sleepiness during the day or close to bed: the stress to sleep. The first sign of sleep being on course is sleep pressure. Sleep stress is your buddy and nothing more than tinkering and trying to catch up on weekends interferes with sleep pressure. Bed pressure is reduced by capping and trapping, ensuring that in the afternoon you feel less pressure for bed.

Eliminate or limit caffeine consumption. Caffeine don't mix with sleep. The misuse of caffeinated drinks—like tea, caffeine, and sodas—and certain ingredients (e.g. chocolate) and medical products can make sleeping hard. Some people, however, are more susceptible than others to caffeine. You might be so fragile that even a small cup of coffee in the morning will make resting and sleeping difficult for you. Do not drink any caffeinated beverages afternoon when you have trouble with your sleep. Even in the evening, you may want to reduce or eliminate caffeine entirely. Don't use caffeine, in particular, to boost yourself if you feel tired. Then, walk around the block for five minutes. Use some exercise to shake off drowsiness rather than caffeine.

Exercise regularly. Regular exercise is one of the safest treatments for sleep. Strong workouts help muscles to relax and relax your worry. Exercise can help relieve the stresses of the day and reduce the propensity of your brain to revisit your busy day information. Aerobic exercise lasts twenty minutes or more at lunch or at the late afternoon. Even an early evening 20-minute stroll could help. Nonetheless, stop intensive activity within 3 hours of bedtime because it can over-stimulate the mind and body and make sleep impossible.

Take a hot bath before bedtime. As the body temperature decreases, sleep tends to come. The faster your temperature drops, the sooner sleep comes—everything else is the same. By bathing in a hot bath just before bedtime, you can use this to your benefit to increase the temperature of your skin. A cold shower does not normally work as well as a hot bath since the core body temperature of the water is difficult to get high enough. You know how the increase in your core body temperature can cause sleep if you have a hot tub or jacuzzi.

Set a consistent bedtime and wake time. Go to sleep every day, even on weekends, and get up at the same time. In the night, even if you are sleepy, at the normal time go out of bed and at the average moment, go to sleep. Consistencies in wake and sleep time keeps sleep pressure adequate and prevents the tending to drift later and later in the day for your sleep and wake cycles. In fact, the body and mind prefer to sleep and wake frequently, so try to honor that.

Create a quiet transition. Bedding is a natural way to wind down and warn the brain that sleep has arrived. Turn off all electronic devices one to two hours before you go to sleep because the ambient light from screens impairs the brain's ability to slow and prepare for sleep. Restrict bedroom sleep habits and involve all other' night stealers' in other parts of the household, such as television viewing, work, and telephone speaking. Rather, listen to the music, bathe in or draw from a book or magazine. Try exercises that are closed to your eyes like meditation, attention or savor. Thought about your day and holding it in your heart while savoring. Love the aroma of your lunch in the tasty green apple. Seek the sound of the ball during your tennis game that day when you have a close touch with him. Taste how good it felt when this project was finished or the sounds of the birds wandering that day. Taste is a good way to finish your day and let your body know it's time for rest. But don't make it to bed—no matter what you do—eat, listen, and meditate. It doesn't work! Do it in anticipation of sleep.

Transform your sleep environment. Another way to show your body that it is time to sleep is a comfortable sleep environment. Stay between 65 and 75 degrees Fahrenheit in your bedroom temperature. Remember, sleep arrives when our bodies start to warm, so make sure your bed is hot and comfortable. Sleep may be interrupted in a cold and stuffy house. Insert a light-resistant shade or heavy ribbons, making your room dark or wearing an eye mask. Finally, use a fan to mask your noises or use earplugs.

Good food, moderate exercise, and enough sleep will improve your physical and mental strength and allow you over time to manage your anxiety. Though it is unlikely that your overwhelming anxiety will be eliminated or your anxiety disorder healed, healthy habits will be a significant part of your recovery plan. Only minor changes in the exercise routine can minimize your anxiety symptoms ' intensity and frequency so that you can do what you previously avoided. In addition, maintaining healthy habits will help you keep track once you recover from your anxiety disorder.

Stress Management Techniques For Vagal Tone Enhancement

Stress has a significant impact on the autonomic nervous system, including vagal tone. By adopting effective stress management techniques, we can enhance vagal tone, promote relaxation, and restore balance to the autonomic nervous system. Here are some stress management techniques that can help enhance vagal tone:

Deep Breathing Exercises

Deep breathing exercises can activate the relaxation response and enhance vagal tone. Focus on taking slow, deep breaths, expanding your belly as you inhale, and exhaling fully. This deep breathing stimulates the vagus nerve and promotes a state of calmness and relaxation. Practicing deep breathing exercises for a few minutes each day can have a profound impact on vagal tone and overall stress reduction.

Meditation and Mindfulness

Meditation and mindfulness practices have been shown to improve vagal tone and reduce stress. By focusing your attention on the present moment, you can cultivate a sense of calm and reduce stress responses. Mindfulness meditation involves observing your thoughts and sensations without judgment. Regular practice of meditation and mindfulness can enhance vagal tone, promote relaxation, and increase resilience to stress.

Yoga and Tai Chi

Yoga and Tai Chi are mind-body practices that combine movement, breathwork, and mindfulness. These practices promote relaxation, reduce stress, and enhance vagal tone. Certain yoga poses, such as forward bends, gentle twists, and inversions, stimulate the vagus nerve and activate the parasympathetic nervous system. Tai Chi, with its slow, flowing movements, promotes relaxation and vagal activation. Regular participation in yoga or Tai Chi can improve vagal tone and support stress management.

Exercise and Physical Activity

Regular physical activity is a potent strategy for stress management and improving vagal tone. Participating in aerobic exercises like brisk walking, jogging, swimming, or cycling heightens heart rate variability and activates the parasympathetic nervous system, which includes the vagus nerve. Strive to engage in moderate-intensity exercise for at least thirty mins on most days of the week to reap the stress-reducing advantages and enhance vagal tone.

Social Support and Connection

Social support and connection are crucial for managing stress and enhancing vagal tone. Positive social interactions, spending time with loved ones, and participating in activities that foster connection and belonging promote a sense of safety and relaxation. Engaging in meaningful relationships and seeking social support when needed can positively impact vagal tone and overall well-being.

Laughter and Humor

Laughter and humor have been shown to enhance vagal tone and reduce stress levels. Engaging in activities that bring joy, like watching a funny movie, spending time with funny friends, or practicing laughter yoga, can stimulate the vagus nerve and trigger the release of endorphins, promoting a sense of well-being and relaxation.

Mindful Eating

Mindful eating can contribute to stress reduction and enhance vagal tone. Instead of eating on the go or in a rushed manner, take the time to sit down, savor your meals, and pay attention to the texture, taste and aroma of the food. Eating mindfully promotes relaxation, proper digestion, and the body's ability to recognize satiety cues.

Self-Care Practices

Engaging in self-care practices is essential for managing stress and promoting vagal tone. Take time for activities that nourish and rejuvenate you, such as taking a bath, practicing self-massage, listening to soothing music, or engaging in a hobby you enjoy. These self-care practices can activate the relaxation response and support vagal activation.

Gratitude and Positive Thinking

Cultivating an attitude of gratitude and practicing positive thinking can enhance vagal tone and reduce stress. Every day, set aside some time to think on the things in your life for which you are thankful and to concentrate on the positive parts of your existence. This practice promotes a positive mindset, reduces negative emotions, and supports vagal activation.

Sleep Hygiene

Adequate and restful sleep is vital for managing stress and promoting optimal vagal tone. Establish a regular sleep schedule, create a calming bedtime routine, and ensure a comfortable sleep environment. Prioritize sleep hygiene practices, like evading electronic devices before bed and creating a peaceful ambiance in your bedroom. Good sleep hygiene supports vagal activation and overall well-being.

Chapter 10:

BONUS: Integrating Vagus Nerve Exercises into Daily Life

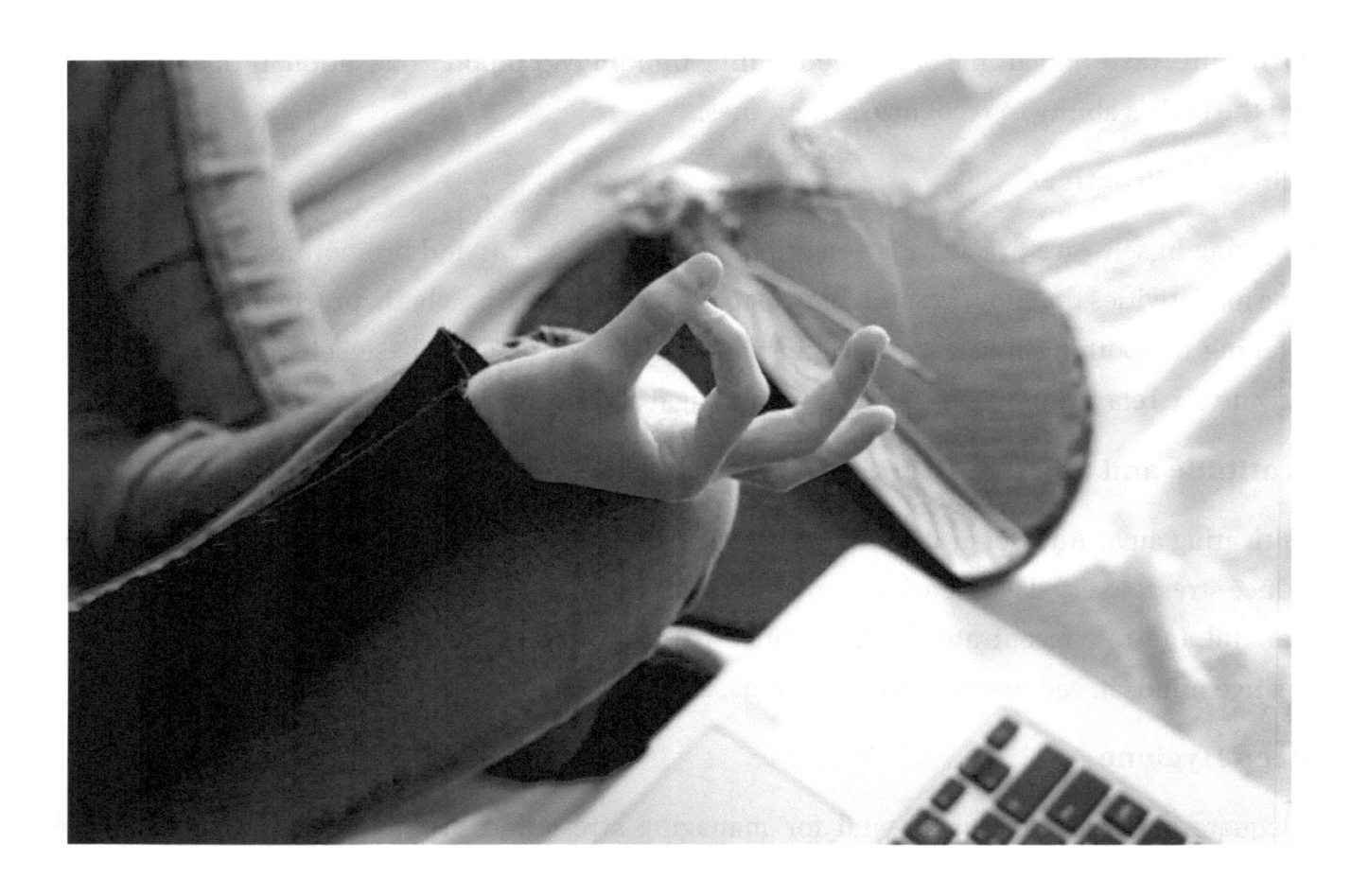

Tips For Incorporating Vagus Nerve Exercises Into A Busy Schedule

Incorporating vagus nerve exercises into a busy schedule can be challenging, but it is essential for promoting relaxation, stress reduction, and overall well-being. By making small adjustments and prioritizing self-care, you can create space for vagus nerve exercises in your daily routine. Here are some tips to help you incorporate these exercises into your busy schedule:

1. Set Clear Intentions: Start by setting clear intentions for incorporating vagus nerve exercises into your daily routine. Recognize the importance of self-care and the benefits

of activating the vagus nerve. Remind yourself that taking care of your well-being is a priority, and commit to making it a part of your daily life.

2. Start with Small Steps: Begin by taking small steps towards incorporating vagus nerve exercises. You should begin with only a couple of mins every day, and as you get more adapted to the activity, you should progressively raise the duration. Remember, consistency is key, even if you can only spare a few minutes each day.

3. Identify Time Blocks: Assess your daily schedule to identify potential time blocks where you can incorporate vagus nerve exercises. It could be in the morning before starting your day, during lunch breaks, in the evening before bed, or any other time that works best for you. Find pockets of time that you can dedicate to these exercises.

4. Make it a Morning Ritual: Consider making vagus nerve exercises a part of your morning ritual. Set aside a few minutes after waking up to engage in deep breathing exercises, meditation, or other practices that stimulate the vagus nerve. Starting your day with these exercises can set a positive tone and promote relaxation throughout the day.

5. Utilize Breaks and Transition Periods: Use breaks and transition periods throughout your day to incorporate vagus nerve exercises. Instead of mindlessly scrolling through your phone or engaging in unproductive activities during breaks, take a few minutes to practice deep breathing, mindfulness, or other exercises. These brief moments can help reset your nervous system and enhance your well-being.

6. Integrate Exercises into Daily Tasks: Look for opportunities to integrate vagus nerve exercises into your daily tasks. For example, while commuting to work or doing household chores, focus on your breath and practice mindful awareness. Use these moments as a chance to engage in deep breathing or other exercises that activate the vagus nerve.

7. Combine Activities: Combine vagus nerve exercises with other activities to maximize your time. For instance, while enjoying a cup of tea or taking a bath, use that time to practice deep breathing or engage in relaxation techniques. This way, you can incorporate self-care into activities you already do, making it more efficient.

8. Create Reminders: Set reminders or alarms on your phone or use sticky notes as visual cues to prompt yourself to engage in vagus nerve exercises. These reminders can help you stay consistent and accountable, especially when you're caught up in a busy schedule.

9. Prioritize Self-Care: Recognize the importance of self-care and prioritize it in your daily schedule. Understand that taking care of your well-being is not a luxury but a necessity.

By making self-care a priority, you'll be more inclined to carve out time for vagus nerve exercises.

10. Flexibility and Adaptability: Be flexible and adaptable with your routine. Some days might be busier than others, and that's okay. If you can't spare the usual amount of time, modify your exercises to fit the available time frame. Even a few minutes of focused breathing or relaxation can have a positive impact.

11. Seek Accountability and Support: Engage in self-care practices with a partner, friend, or family member. Share your goals and progress with someone who can provide accountability and support. You can engage in exercises together or simply check in with each other to ensure you're both prioritizing self-care.

12. Be Gentle with Yourself: Remember to be gentle with yourself and avoid self-judgment. There may be days when you are unable to follow your routine or complete the exercises as planned. It's important to accept that setbacks happen and that self-care is a journey. Offer yourself compassion and get back on track when you can.

Strategies For Maintaining Consistency And Motivation

Maintaining consistency and motivation in any practice, including vagus nerve exercises, can be challenging. However, by implementing effective strategies, you can overcome obstacles and stay committed to your self-care routine. Here are some strategies for maintaining consistency and motivation:

1. Set Clear Goals: Start by setting clear and realistic goals for your vagus nerve exercises. Define what you want to achieve and why it is important to you. Having a clear purpose will keep you focused and motivated. Make sure your goals are specific, measurable, achievable, relevant, and time-bound (SMART goals).

2. Create a Routine: Establishing a regular routine is crucial for maintaining consistency. Choose specific times during the day when you will dedicate to your vagus nerve exercises. Consistency helps build habits and makes it easier to follow through even on busy days. Treat these exercises as non-negotiable appointments with yourself.

3. Track Your Progress: Keep track of your progress to stay motivated and see the positive impact of your efforts. Use a journal, a mobile app, or any other method that works for

you to record your daily practice. Seeing your progress can be inspiring and reinforce your commitment.

4. Find Accountability: Find an accountability partner or join a supportive community to keep you motivated. Share your goals and progress with someone who can hold you accountable. It could be a friend, family member, or an online group. Knowing that someone is expecting you to follow through can provide the necessary motivation to stay consistent.

5. Celebrate Milestones: Celebrate your milestones along the way. Acknowledge and reward yourself for your achievements, no matter how small they may seem. Treat yourself to something you enjoy or engage in a self-care activity as a way of recognizing your commitment and progress.

6. Mix Up Your Exercises: Keep your routine fresh and engaging by incorporating a variety of vagus nerve exercises. Explore different techniques such as deep breathing, meditation, yoga, chanting, or sound therapy. Trying new exercises can help prevent monotony and maintain your interest and motivation.

7. Make it Enjoyable: Find ways to make your vagus nerve exercises enjoyable. Listen to calming music or guided meditations, practice in a serene environment, or personalize your routine to suit your preferences. When you enjoy the practice, you are more likely to look forward to it and maintain consistency.

8. Be Flexible and Adapt: Life can be unpredictable, and there may be days when it's challenging to stick to your routine. Be flexible and adapt to these situations. If you're short on time, modify your exercises or break them into smaller sessions throughout the day. The key is to find ways to continue the practice, even in a modified form.

9. Focus on the Benefits: Remind yourself of the benefits you experience from your vagus nerve exercises. Reflect on how these exercises contribute to your well-being, stress reduction, and overall quality of life. When you recognize the positive impact, it serves as a powerful motivator to maintain consistency.

10. Practice Self-Compassion: Practice self-kindness and compassion, treating yourself with gentleness and understanding. If you miss a day or struggle to maintain consistency, don't beat yourself up. Accept that setbacks happen, and it's part of the journey. Treat yourself with understanding and self-compassion, and use it as an opportunity to recommit and continue moving forward.

11. Seek Inspiration: Surround yourself with inspiration and motivation. Read books, watch videos or listen to podcasts related to vagus nerve exercises and self-care. Engage in activities that uplift and inspire you. Seek out stories of others who have benefited from these practices to reignite your motivation.

12. Reflect on the Positive Effects: Take time to reflect on the positive effects of your vagus nerve exercises in your daily life. Notice how you feel more relaxed, centered, and resilient. Pay attention to improvements in your stress levels, sleep quality, emotional well-being, and overall health. Cultivate a sense of gratitude for the positive changes these exercises bring.

Tracking Progress And Observing The Benefits Of Regular Practice

Tracking progress and observing the benefits of regular practice is an important aspect of any self-care routine, including vagus nerve exercises. Not only does it provide motivation and a sense of accomplishment, but it also allows you to make informed adjustments and witness the positive impact these exercises have on your overall well-being. Here are some reasons why tracking progress and observing the benefits of regular practice is essential, along with practical ways to do so:

1. **Motivation and Accountability**

Tracking progress serves as a source of motivation and accountability. When you see tangible evidence of your efforts, it reinforces your commitment to the practice. It helps you stay focused and reminds you of the positive changes you are working towards.

Practical Tip: Keep a journal or a dedicated notebook where you can record your daily practice. Note down the duration, specific exercises or techniques you used, and any observations or reflections. This will help you see the progress you are making over time.

2. **Self-Awareness and Reflection**

Observing the benefits of regular practice allows you to develop self-awareness and reflect on the changes happening within yourself. By paying attention to how you feel physically, mentally, and emotionally, you can better understand the impact of vagus nerve exercises on your overall well-being.

Practical Tip: Take a few moments after each practice to sit quietly and tune into your body and mind. Observe any shifts or sensations you experience. Notice changes in your stress levels, mood, energy, or any other aspects of your well-being. Write down your observations in your journal to track patterns and progress.

3. Identifying Patterns and Adjustments

Tracking progress helps you identify patterns and make adjustments to your practice as needed. By noting the frequency, duration, and techniques used, you can analyze what works best for you and make informed decisions about refining your routine.

Practical Tip: Review your journal regularly and look for patterns or trends. Are there particular exercises that consistently leave you feeling more relaxed? Do you notice any patterns in your stress levels throughout the week? Use this information to adjust your practice accordingly. You may choose to allocate more time to certain exercises or experiment with new techniques.

4. Reinforcing Positive Habits

Regularly observing the benefits of your practice reinforces positive habits. As you witness the positive impact on your well-being, you become more motivated to continue the practice and integrate it into your daily life as a habit.

Practical Tip: Create a visual representation of your progress. For example, use a habit tracker or a calendar to mark the days you engaged in vagus nerve exercises. Seeing a string of consistent practice can be visually rewarding and serve as a reminder of your commitment.

5. Enhancing Mindfulness and Presence

Tracking progress and observing benefits encourages mindfulness and presence during your practice. When you actively pay attention to the effects of each exercise, you cultivate a deeper connection with your body, mind, and emotions.

Practical Tip: During your practice, bring a sense of curiosity and mindfulness to each technique. Notice the physical sensations, the rhythm of your breath, and the thoughts that arise. Allow yourself to fully experience the present moment. This level of mindfulness enhances the benefits of vagus nerve exercises and deepens your awareness of their impact.

6. Celebrating Milestones and Progress

Observing the benefits of regular practice allows you to celebrate milestones and acknowledge your progress. It's important to recognize and celebrate even the small victories along the way, as they contribute to your overall well-being.

Practical Tip: Set mini-goals or milestones for yourself and celebrate each one you achieve. It could be completing a certain number of consecutive days of practice, increasing the duration of your exercises, or noticing specific positive changes. Celebrate these milestones in a way that is meaningful to you, such as treating yourself to something you enjoy or engaging in a self-care activity.

7. Self-Empowerment and Self-Care Advocacy

Tracking progress and observing the benefits of regular practice empowers you to take charge of your own well-being. It reinforces the idea that you have the ability to make positive changes in your life and that self-care is a vital aspect of your overall health.

Practical Tip: Share your progress and experiences with others who might benefit from vagus nerve exercises or self-care practices. By advocating for self-care, you not only reinforce your own commitment but also inspire others to prioritize their well-being.

Chapter 11:

Glossary of Terms

Affirmations: Positive statements or phrases that are repeated to promote positive thinking and shift mindset. Using affirmations that promote self-love, relaxation, and gratitude can enhance vagal tone and cultivate a positive outlook.

Autonomic Nervous System: The part of the peripheral nervous system that is in charge of regulating involuntary actions of the body, such as the rate at which the heart beats, digestion, and breathing.

Diaphragmatic Breathing: A breathing technique that involves deep inhalation and exhalation using the diaphragm muscle. It promotes relaxation, activates the parasympathetic nervous system, and enhances vagal tone.

Guided Imagery: A relaxation technique that involves guided visualization to create mental images and promote a state of calm. Guided imagery activates the vagus nerve and can be used for stress reduction and relaxation.

Heart Rate Variability (HRV): Variability in the length of time that elapses amongst successive beating of the heart. Higher HRV is associated with better vagal tone and overall cardiovascular health.

Meditation: A practice that comprises training the mind to focus and redirect thoughts, often through techniques such as mindfulness or visualization. Meditation can enhance vagus nerve activity and promote relaxation.

Mind-Body Connection: The relationship and interaction between the mind (thoughts, emotions) and the body (physiology, sensations). Cultivating a strong mind-body connection through vagus nerve exercises promotes overall well-being.

Neuroplasticity: The capacity of the brain to adapt to new information and restructure itself during one's lifetime as a result of situations, learning, and the influence of the surrounding environment. Vagus nerve exercises can enhance neuroplasticity and support brain health.

Self-Regulation: The ability to regulate one's thoughts, emotions, and behaviors in response to internal and external stimuli. Vagus nerve exercises help improve self-regulation skills, leading to better emotional well-being.

Sound Healing: The therapeutic use of sound vibrations to promote relaxation, reduce stress, and restore balance in the body and mind. Sound healing practices, such as chanting or using specific frequencies, can stimulate the vagus nerve.

Stress Reduction: Techniques, practices, and strategies aimed at reducing the physiological and psychological effects of stress on the body. Vagus nerve exercises play a significant role in stress reduction and promoting relaxation.

Tai Chi: A traditional form of martial arts practiced in China that emphasizes slowness, fluidity, and concentration through the use of deep breathing and flowing movements. Tai Chi promotes relaxation, improves balance, and enhances vagal tone.

Vagal Maneuvers: Physical techniques used to stimulate the vagus nerve and regulate heart rate. Examples include the Valsalva maneuver, carotid sinus massage, and cold water face immersion.

Vagus Nerve Stimulation (VNS): A medical procedure that involves the use of an implanted device to deliver electrical impulses to the vagus nerve. VNS has been used to treat certain neurological and psychiatric conditions.

Well-being: A state of physical, mental, and emotional health characterized by a sense of balance, contentment, and vitality. Regular vagus nerve exercises contribute to overall well-being and enhance the mind-body connection.

Yoga: A comprehensive practice that integrates physical postures, the management of one's breath, the act of meditation, and ethical precepts. Yoga can activate the parasympathetic nervous system, increase vagal tone, and promote relaxation and well-being.

Yogic Breathing Techniques: Pranayama practices in yoga that involve specific breath control techniques. These techniques, such as alternate nostril breathing or belly breathing, can enhance vagal tone and induce relaxation.

Conclusion

Understanding and nurturing the health of the vagus nerve is essential for promoting overall well-being and maintaining a balanced mind-body connection. The vagus nerve, with its intricate network of connections throughout the body, plays a vital role in regulating various bodily functions and influencing our physical and mental health.

By incorporating daily vagus nerve exercises, such as deep breathing, yoga, sound therapy, physical activity, massage, and a healthy lifestyle, we can actively stimulate and support the function of the vagus nerve. These practices have numerous benefits, including stress reduction and relaxation, improved digestion and gut health, enhanced immune system function, emotional regulation, and increased resilience.

It's essential to remember that vagus nerve health is a lifelong journey, and consistency is key. Making these exercises and practices a regular part of our daily routine can yield long-term benefits. To support your commitment to lifelong vagus nerve health, here are some final thoughts and words of encouragement:

- Start small and be patient: Incorporating vagus nerve exercises into your daily routine may take time and practice. Begin with simple techniques and carefully elevate their duration or intensity as you become more comfortable. Embrace the process and be patient with yourself.
- Find what resonates with you: There are various techniques available for vagus nerve activation, so explore different practices and find what resonates with you. Experiment with different breathwork techniques, yoga styles, or sound therapy approaches to discover what brings you the most relaxation and stress relief.
- Create a routine: Establishing a consistent routine is essential for reaping the long-term benefits of vagus nerve exercises. Set aside dedicated time each day to engage in these practices, even if it's just for a few minutes. Consistency is key to forming a habit and experiencing the cumulative effects of vagus nerve activation.
- Stay mindful and present: Mindfulness is a powerful tool for enhancing the mind-body connection. As you engage in vagus nerve exercises, cultivate a sense of mindfulness and presence. Focus on the sensations, thoughts, and emotions that arise during these practices. This heightened awareness can deepen the benefits and bring a greater sense of calm and balance to your daily life.
- Seek support and guidance: If you're new to vagus nerve exercises or need additional guidance, consider seeking support from professionals or experienced practitioners. Yoga

instructors, meditation teachers, therapists, or healthcare providers can offer valuable insights and help tailor practices to your specific needs and goals.
- Celebrate progress and observe the benefits: Take time to reflect on your journey and observe the positive changes that occur as you prioritize vagus nerve health. Notice improvements in stress levels, digestion, immune function, emotional well-being, and overall resilience. Celebrate your progress, no matter how small, and use it as motivation to continue your commitment to lifelong vagus nerve health.

Remember, the journey to vagus nerve health is unique to each individual. Listen to your body, honor its needs, and adapt your practices accordingly. Embrace the interconnectedness of the mind and body and prioritize self-care as a means to nurture and support your vagus nerve health.

With consistent effort and a holistic approach, you can cultivate a lifelong practice of vagus nerve exercises that supports your well-being, resilience, and overall vitality. Embrace the power of the vagus nerve and its ability to promote balance, relaxation, and optimal health in your life.

If you have read this book, I would greatly appreciate your feedback and review. Your review will help me understand the strengths and areas for improvement, allowing me to enhance the book and provide a better experience for readers. Thank you for your time and valuable input!